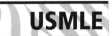 

BEHAVIORAL SCIENCES AND OUTPATIENT MEDICINE

for the
Boards and Wards

Other books in the Boards and Wards series:

Boards and Wards — USMLE Steps 2 and 3
Pathophysiology for the Boards and Wards — USMLE Step 1
Dermatology for the Boards and Wards — USMLE Review
Immunology for the Boards and Wards — USMLE Step 1
Ophthalmology/ENT for the Boards and Wards — USMLE Steps 1, 2, and 3
Microbiology for the Boards and Wards — USMLE Step 1

BEHAVIORAL SCIENCES AND OUTPATIENT MEDICINE

for the
Boards and Wards

Carlos Ayala, MD
Clinical Fellow in Otology and Laryngology
Harvard Medical School
Resident in Otolaryngology
Harvard Otolaryngology Residency Program
Boston, Massachussetts

Brad Spellberg, MD
Resident in Internal Medicine
Harbor-UCLA Medical Center
Torrance, California

Blackwell
Science

©2001 by Carlos Ayala and Brad Spellberg

Editorial Offices:
Commerce Place, 350 Main Street, Malden, Massachusetts 02148, USA
Osney Mead, Oxford OX2 0EL, England
25 John Street, London WC1N 2BL, England
23 Ainslie Place, Edinburgh EH3 6AJ, Scotland
54 University Street, Carlton, Victoria 3053, Australia

Other Editorial Offices:
Blackwell Wissenschafts-Verlag GmbH, Kurfürstendamm 57, 10707 Berlin, Germany
Blackwell Science KK, MG Kodenmacho Building, 7-10 Kodenmacho Nihombashi,
   Chuo-ku, Tokyo 104, Japan
Iowa State University Press, A Blackwell Science Company, 2121 S. State Avenue, Ames,
   Iowa 50014-8300, USA

Distributors:

USA
Blackwell Science, Inc.
Commerce Place
350 Main Street
Malden, Massachusetts 02148
(Telephone orders: 800-215-1000 or
   781-388-8250; fax orders: 781-388-8270)

Canada
Login Brothers Book Company
324 Saulteaux Crescent
Winnipeg, Manitoba R3J 3T2
(Telephone orders: 204-837-2987)

Australia
Blackwell Science Pty, Ltd.
54 University Street
Carlton, Victoria 3053
(Telephone orders: 03-9347-0300;
   fax orders: 03-9349-3016)

Outside North America and Australia
Blackwell Science, Ltd.
c/o Marston Book Services, Ltd.
P.O. Box 269
Abingdon
Oxon OX14 4YN
England
(Telephone orders: 44-01235-465500;
   fax orders: 44-01235-465555)

Acquisitions: Beverly Copland
Development: Julia Casson
Production: Irene Herlihy
Manufacturing: Lisa Flanagan

Marketing Manager: Toni Fournier
Typeset by Software Services
Printed and bound by Capital City Press

Printed in the United States of America
01 02 03 04 5 4 3 2 1

Library of Congress Cataloging-in-Publication Data
Ayala, Carlos, MD.
   Behavioral sciences and outpatient medicine for the boards and wards/by Carlos Ayala
   and Brad Spellberg.
      p.; cm.
   ISBN 0-632-04578-7
   1. Social medicine—Examinations, questions, etc. 2. Ambulatory medical
   care—Examinations, questions, etc. 3. Medicine, Preventive—Examinations, questions,
   etc. 4. Psychiatry—Examinations, questions, etc. I. Spellberg, Brad. II. Title.
   [DNLM: 1. Behavioral Sciences—Examination Questions. 2. Ambulatory
   Care—psychology—Examination Questions. WM 18.2 A973b 2001]
   RA418 .A96 2001
   610'.76—dc21
                                                                    2001025023

TABLE OF CONTENTS

Tables   vii

Abbreviations   ix

Preface   xi

Acknowledgments   xiii

I.   Doctoring   1

II.   Health Care Delivery   5

III.   Growth and Development   7

IV.   Child and Adolescent Medicine   10

V.   Child and Adolescent Psychiatry   14

VI.   Drugs of Abuse   18

VII.   Psychiatry/Mood Disorders   19

VIII.   Psychosis   23

IX.   Anxiety Disorders   26

X.   Personality Disorders   28

XI.   Somatoform and Factitious Disorders   30

XII.   Miscellaneous Disorders   33

XIII.   Sleep   35

XIV. Nutrition   37

XV. Toxicology   41

XVI. Common Outpatient Complaints and
Treatments   46

XVII. Common Sports Medicine Complaints   70

XVIII. Preventive Medicine   75

XIX. Law and Ethics   78

XX. Biostatistics   80

Review Questions   83

Answers   87

Index   89

TABLES

1 Interviewing Techniques   2

2 Developmental Theories   7

3 Developmental Milestones   8

4 Tanner Stages   9

5 Psychological Tests   9

6 Pediatric Toxicology   13

7 Drug Intoxications and Withdrawal   19

8 DSM-IV Classification   20

9 Prognosis of Psychiatric Disorders   20

10 Mood Disorders   21

11 Pharmacologic Therapy for Depression   22

12 Diagnosis of Psychotic Disorders   23

13 Antipsychotic Drugs   24

14 Antipsychotic Associated Movements Disorders   25

15 Anxiety Disorders   26

16 Specific Personality Disorders   29

17 Dementia versus Delerium   35

18 Sleep Stages   36

19 Vitamins and Minerals   40

20 Toxicology   42

21 Fish and Shellfish Toxins   44

22 Bites and Stings   45

23 Summary of Headaches   47

24 Treatment of Headaches   48

25 Sinusitis   49

26 Pharyngitis   50

27 Diarrhea   53

28 Infectious Causes of Diarrhea   55

29 Sexually Transmitted Diseases   56

30 Differential Diagnosis of Vaginitis   65

31 Low Back Pain Red Flags   72

32 Cancer Screening   76

33 Adult Immunization   76

34 Travel Prophylaxis   77

35 Tetanus Immunization   78

36 Biostatistics and Epidemiology   81

37 Sample Calculation of Statistical Values   83

ABBREVIATIONS

↑ (↑↑)	increases/high (markedly increases/very high)
↓ (↓↓)	decreases/low (markedly decreases/very low)
→	causes/leads to/analysis shows
1°/2°	primary/secondary
BP	blood pressure
Bx	biopsy
CA	carcinoma
CN	cranial nerve
CNS	central nervous system
CXR/X-ray	chest x-ray/x-ray
Dx/DDx	diagnosis/differential diagnosis
ETOH	ethyl alcohol
dz	disease
HA	headache
HTN	hypertension
Hx/FHx	history/family history
ICP	intracranial pressure
I&D	incision and drainage
infxn	infection
IVIG	intravenous immunoglobulin
N or Nml	normal
PE	physical exam or pulmonary embolus
pt(s)	patient(s)
Px	prognosis
Si/Sx/aSx	sign/symptom/asymptomatic
subQ	subcutaneous
Tx	treatment/therapy
Utz	ultrasound

PREFACE

This book was designed for hardworking medical students and residents who must pass the Boards to practice as licensed physicians on the Wards. A common theme in all our books is the presentation of only the necessary information in a clinically relevent, concise manner.

One of the topics addressed on all three steps of the USMLE is Behavioral Sciences. This grab-bag term encompasses many subjects, such as statistics, preventive medicine, health maintenance, law, ethics, psychiatry, and common outpatient complaints.

We bring you the key points in Behavioral Sciences most frequently asked on the USMLE in a quick and concise fashion. We also include many of the topics not addressed by other similar review books on the market and not addressed in classes at most medical schools. We discuss topics such as cultural medicine, toxicology, nutrition, sports, and travel medicine. No other book on the market so broadly addresses the needs of those taking the USMLE Steps 1–3 in such a concise manner.

We hope you find this book useful to you on the Boards and Wards.

ACKNOWLEDGMENTS

Special thanks to Charles Lee, Beatriz Mares, Griselda Gutierrez, and Pedro Cheung, whose previous work on Boards and Wards Steps 2 and 3 inspired and assisted in the completion of this new project.

I. DOCTORING

A. Introduction

1. Patient–Doctor (physician) relationship is based on trust, confidence, mutual understanding, and communication
2. Patient interviews and interactions must be conducted in a humanistic, culturally sensitive manner
3. In cooperation with other health care professionals, such as interpreters, an appreciation for racial and cultural diversity must always be conveyed
4. Non-biased health care delivery to the patient and their family must be conveyed at all times
5. Treatment plans must be realistic, mutually understood, and mutually agreed upon to achieve compliance

B. Interview

1. Introduce self to patient; assure an interpreter is present if a foreign language is spoken
2. Face patient, and always speak to patient and their family directly and not to the interpreter
3. Try not to interrupt patient when speaking
4. Interviewing techniques (Table 1)
5. Patient history: chief complaint, history of present illness (HPI), past medical history (PMH), past surgical history (PSH), family history (FH), social history (SH) and allergies
6. Helpful interviewing mnemonic (**HEADSSS**)

   a. Originally developed to interview adolescents but can be used for all ages as a way to break the ice of an initial interview and to cover major areas

   b. **HEADSSS** assessment allows physicians to evaluate critical areas in each patient's life that may be detrimental to their health

      1) **H**ome environment: Who does patient live with? Any recent changes? Quality of family interaction (if applicable)?

      2) **H**ealth risks: Exposure to TB, Hepatitis, asbestos, cigarette smoke, radiation

TABLE 1	Interviewing Techniques	
TECHNIQUE	**DESCRIPTION**	**EXAMPLE**
Empathy	Communicating an understanding of patient's feelings.	"I can tell you must really be upset about this situation."
Paraphrasing	Communicates an understanding of content.	"So you have been waiting three hours for your appointment."
Silence	A pause in a conversation is worth a thousand words. Doctor and patient can use this time to watch each other's nonverbal posturing and to take an inventory of how interview is going.	"-----------------------------"
Open-ended questions	Allows patient and family to express themselves fully regarding the topic in question.	"Why have you come to the hospital today?"
Questions for the doctor	Allow patient to express their concerns and to assure themselves of what has been discussed during the interview and what still has not been addressed.	"Do you have any questions for me?"
Direct questioning	Allows the interviewer to focus on an important topic.	"Now tell me more about how you got that bruise on your arm."
Identifying/ validation	Allows patient's concerns to appear acceptable and worth discussing.	"I am also afraid of doctors and hospitals; please tell me more about why you are here."

3) Employment and Education: Is patient in school? Favorite subjects? Academic performance? Are friends in school? Any recent changes? Does patient have a job? Future plans?

4) Activities: What does patient like to do in spare time? Who does patient spend time with? Involved in any sports/exercise? Hobbies? Attends parties or clubs?

5) Drugs: Has patient ever used tobacco? Alcohol? Marijuana? Other illicit drugs? If so, when was the last use? How often? Do friends or family members use drugs? Who does the patient use these substances with?

6) Sexual activity: Sexual orientation? Is patient sexually active? Number of sexual partners? Does the patient use condoms or other forms of contraception? Any history of STDs or pregnancy?

7) Suicide: Does the patient ever feel sad, tired, or unmotivated? Has the patient ever felt that life was not worth living? Any feelings of wanting to harm self? If so, does the patient have a plan? Has the patient ever tried to harm self in the past? Does the patient know anyone who has attempted suicide?

8) Safety: Does the patient use a seat belt or bike helmet? Does the patient enter into high-risk situations? Does the patient have access to a firearm? Is the patient's home environment safe?

C. Identifying Abuse

1. Not necessarily physical in nature. Can be physical assault, sexual assault, psychological abuse, economic control and/or progressive social isolation

2. Depending on state laws, certain potential abuse situations mandate reporting. Failure to report subjects practitioner to disciplinary action, fines, and/or liability

3. Department of Social Services should be made aware of suspected child abuse and elder abuse cases

4. Cameras and rape kits should made available in all emergency departments to properly handle potential evidence

5. Must know and understand cultural demographics of community served. Certain cultural medicine rituals may be misinterpreted by health practitioners

   a. Cupping: Cupping, pinching, or rubbing (also known as coining). Thought to restore balance by releasing excessive "air"

      1) Small cups are used, small shot glasses. A small amount of alcohol is put into the cup and ignited, and the cup is immediately pressed tight against the skin (forehead, abdomen, chest, or back). A vacuum is produced by the combustion of the alcohol and the evacuation of oxygen from the cup. The developing vacuum then sucks out noxious materials or excess energy into the cup from the body. A circular ecchymotic area is left on the skin

b. Pinching: Pressure is applied by pinching the skin between the thumb and index finger to the point of producing a contusion. Done at the base of the nose, between the eyes, on the neck, chest, or back

c. Rubbing is usually in the same areas as pinching and involves firmly rubbing lubricated skin with a spoon or a coin in order to bring toxic "air" to the body surface

d. Female genital mutilation carried out today in more than 30 countries across Africa and the Middle East. Awareness of this practice and its consequences is necessary to adequately treat these patients

D. Cultural Medicine

1. Hot & Cold theory: Seen in Latin American cultures; illness is caused by an imbalance of hot and cold. Eating appropriately hot or cold type foods as needed can restore balance

2. Prominent among Mexican–American folk healers is the curandero, a type of shaman who uses white magic and herbs to effect cures

3. Five types of folk illness are most prominent:

   a. mal de ojo (evil eye)

   b. empacho (gastro-intestinal blockage due to excessive food intake)

   c. susto (magically induced fright)

   d. caida de la mollera (fallen fontanel, or opening in or between bones)

   e. mal puesto (sorcery)

E. Interpreter

1. In order to provide best available patient services, all efforts should be made to facilitate communications with patient in their language, using an interpreter whenever possible

2. Physician must always face patient and speak directly to patient while discussion is translated

3. Have patient repeat instructions to you through interpreter to assure understanding

4. Whenever possible use a trained interpreter and avoid using family members to prevent embarrassment, and miscommunication of discussion

II. HEALTH CARE DELIVERY

A. Hospitals

1. Tertiary Medical Center: Receives referrals from community, has latest technologies, including organ transplantation, Level 1 trauma, etc. Most academic medical centers

2. Intermediate Hospital: No organ transplantation, much of the same technology as a major medical center

3. Community Hospital: Provides basic services, lacks major staffing and technology of larger medical centers

B. Health Maintenance Organizations (HMOs)

1. Provide health care to people who have prepaid enrollment

2. Various models exist: Staff Model, Preferred Provider Organization (PPO), and Independent Practice Association (IPA)

   a. Staff Model: Physicians are salaried employees or contracted to provide medical services to members. All patients must be seen by a primary care physician prior to referral to most specialists

   b. PPOs: Occurs when an insurance company has established contracts with certain independent providers, allowing patients to choose physicians not normally on their list of providers for a surcharge

   c. IPAs: Physicians paid on an agreed upon fee-for-service whenever a member of the HMO uses their services

3. Capitation: Physicians are paid a certain amount per patient, per year, regardless of the amount of services provided to each of the patients assigned

C. Extended Care Facilities

1. Nursing homes/skilled nursing facilities (SNFs)

   a. Provide intravenous fluids, nutrition, and medications

   b. Nursing staff available 24 hr

2. Intermediate care facilities (ICF)

    a. Provide assistance mainly with activities of daily living

    b. Nursing not necessarily available 24 hr

D. Hospice

1. Specializes in providing terminal care to patients in their final moments of life

E. Medicare/Medicaid

1. Medicare: Authorized under the Social Security Act

    a. Provides health insurance to people over 65 years old or who are disabled and receive social security, does *not* cover prescription medications

2. Medicaid: Also authorized under the Social Security Act

    a. Unlike Medicare, it is provided to the very poor who usually receive other types of public assistance. Qualifications vary by state, does cover prescription medications

F. Hospital Personnel

1. Nurses: Many levels of training

    a. Nurse's Aid: Basic medical vocational training

    b. LPN/LVN: Licensed Practical Nurse/Licensed Vocational Nurse, undergo a 1 yr program of nursing vocational training followed by a state licensing exam

    c. Registered Nurse: May have a Bachelors degree or Associate degree, have passed state nursing board exams and have a registered state license

    d. Clinical Nurse Specialist: Usually Masters degree prepared nurse, has advanced training in a specific medical area, i.e., intensive care, cardiac care, enterostomal care, etc.

    e. Nurse Practitioner: Usually Masters degree prepared nurse, practice as a family nurse practitioner, pediatric nurse practitioner, nursing midwife

    f. Doctoral Nurses: Hold Doctorate degree in various areas, mainly work in academic nursing schools as professors and researchers

  2. Physician Assistant: Usually Bachelors degree level of education, and a state licensing exam. Function as independent practitioners under the supervision of a physician

III. GROWTH AND DEVELOPMENT

A. Developmental Theories (Table 2)

TABLE 2	Developmental Theories			
AGE (YEARS)	**FREUD**	**ERICKSON**	**PIAGET**	**MAJOR THEME**
0–1	**Oral** Everything goes in mouth	**Trust vs. Mistrust** Child trusts all basic needs to be met.	**Sensorimotor** Mastery of environment (0–2 yr)	**Stranger Anxiety** Immense anxiety when separated from mother, between 6 and 9 mo.
1–3	**Anal** Toilet training	**Autonomy vs. Shame and Doubt**	**Preoperational** Symbolic terms (2–7 yr)	**Separation Anxiety** (18 mo–3 yr)
3–5	**Phallic-oedipal**	**Initiative vs. Guilt**	**Preoperational**	**Imaginary Friends**
6–11	**Latency**	**Industry vs. Inferiority**	**Concrete Operations** (7–11 yr)	**Logical Thoughts**
11–20	**Genital**	**Identity vs. Difusion**	**Formal Operations**	**Abstract Thoughts**
20–40		**Intimacy vs. Isolation**		
40–65		**Generativity vs. Stagnation**		
>65		**Ego Integrity vs. Despair**		

B. Developmental Milestones (Table 3)

TABLE 3	**Developmental Milestones**			
AGE (MONTHS)	**GROSS MOTOR**	**FINE MOTOR**	**LANGUAGE**	**SOCIAL/ COGNITION**
Newborn	Head side to side, **Moro & grasp reflex**			
2	Holds head up	Swipes at object	Coos	Social smile
4	Rolls front to back	**Grasps object**	Orients to voice	Laughs
6	Rolls back to front, **sits upright**	Transfers object	Babbles	**Stranger anxiety, sleeps all night**
9	Crawls, pulls to stand	**Pincer grasp,** eats with fingers	**Mama-dada (nonspecific)**	Waves bye-bye, responds to name
12	**Stands**	**Mature pincer**	**Mama-dada (specific)**	Picture book
15	**Walks**	Uses cup	4–6 words	**Temper tantrum**
18	Throws ball, walks upstairs	Uses spoon for solids	Names common objects	**Toilet training may begin**
24	Runs, up/down stairs	Uses spoon for semisolids	**2-word sentence** (2 word at 2 yr)	Follows 2-step command
36	Rides tricycle	Eats neatly with utensils	**3-word sentence** (3 word at 3 yr)	Knows first & last name

C. Tanner Stages (Table 4)

TABLE 4	Tanner Stages	
BOYS	**GIRLS**
Testicular enlargement at 11.5 yr*	Breast buds at 10.5 yr*
Increase in genital size	Pubic hair
Pubic hair	Linear growth spurt at 12 yr
Peak growth spurt at 13.5 yr*	Menarche at 12.5 yr*
*Years represent population averages.	

D. Psychological Tests (Table 5)

TABLE 5	Psychological Tests	
INTELLIGENCE	
Wechsler Adult Intelligence Scale—Revised (WAIS-R)	Tests ability to reason new situations, and assimilate, organize, and process this information. Tests cover verbal comprehension, performance at picture completion, block design, etc.
Wechsler Intelligence Scale for Children—Revised (WISC-R)	Tests children 6–16
Wechsler Preschool and Primary Scale of Intelligence (WPPSI)	Tests children 4–6
PERSONALITY	
Minnesota Multiphasic Personality Inventory (MMPI)	Most common objective personality test. Determines personality type.
Rorschach	Most common projective test. Ink blot designs are interpreted, and defense mechanisms and thought disorders are evaluated
ACHIEVEMENT	
Wide-Range Achievement Test (WRAT)	Evaluates content-specific knowledge. Topics include spelling, reading, math, and science.

IV. CHILD AND ADOLESCENT MEDICINE

A. Trauma and Intoxication

1. Child abuse

   a. Can be physical trauma, emotional, sexual, or neglect

   b. Nutritional neglect is the most common etiology for underweight infants

   c. Most common perpetrator of sexual abuse is family member or family friends, 97% of reported offenders are males

   d. **Physicians are required by law to report suspected child abuse or neglect (law provides protection to mandated reporters who report in good faith), clinical & lab evaluations are allowed without parental/guardian permission**

   e. Epidemiology

      1) Eighty-five percent of children reported to children's protective services (CPS) are <5 yr old, 45% are <1 yr old

      2) Ten percent of injuries to children <5 yr old seen in the ER are due to abuse, and 10% of abuse cases involve burns

      3) **High-risk children** = premature infants, children with chronic medical problems, colicky babies, those with behavioral problems, children living in poverty, children of teenage parents, single parents, or substance abusers

   f. Si/Sx = injury is unexplainable or not consistent with Hx, bruises are the most common manifestation

      1) Accidental injuries seen on shins, forearms, hips

      2) Less likely to be accidental are bilateral & symmetric, seen on buttocks, genitalia, back, back of hands, different color bruises (repeat injuries over time)

      3) Highly suspicious for abuse are fractures due to pulling or wrenching, causing damage to the metaphysis

   g. **Classic findings**

      1) Chip fracture, where the corner of metaphysis of long bone is torn off with damage to epiphysis

2) Periosteum spiral fracture before infant can walk

3) Rib fractures

h. Dating fracture can be done by callus formation (callus appears in 10–12 days)

i. Burns

1) Shape/pattern of burn may be diagnostic

2) **Cigarette** → circular, punched out lesions of similar size, hands and feet common

3) **Immersion** → most common in infants, affecting buttocks and perineum (hold thighs against abdomen), or with scalded line clearly demarcated on thighs or waist without splash marks, stocking-glove burn on hands or feet

j. Injury to head is the most common cause of death from physical abuse, infants can present with convulsions, apnea, increased intracranial pressure, subdural hemorrhages, retinal hemorrhages (marker for acceleration/deceleration injuries), or in a coma

k. Sexual abuse

1) Child may talk to mother or teacher, friend, relative about situation

2) Si/Sx = vaginal, penile, or rectal pain, erythema, discharge, bleeding, chronic dysuria, enuresis, constipation, encopresis

3) Behaviors = sexualized activity with peers or objects, seductive behavior

l. Dx

1) Labs → PT/PTT & platelets to screen for bleeding diathesis

2) Consider bone survey in children <2 yr old, plain films or MRI for severe injuries, or refusal/inability to communicate

3) For sexual abuse, collect specimens of offender's sperm, blood, & hair, collect victim's nail clipping & clothing, obtain *Chlamydia* & gonorrhea cultures from mouth, anus, & genitalia

4) Dx is tentatively based on H&P, record all information, and photograph when appropriate

m. Tx

    1) Medical, surgical, psychiatric treatment for injuries

    2) Report immediately, do not discharge before talking to CPS

    3) Admit pt if injuries are severe enough, if Dx unclear, or if no other safe placement available

2. Poisonings

    a. Accidental seen in younger children left unsupervised momentarily, usually a single agent ingested or inhaled (plants, household products, medications)

    b. Intentional seen in adolescents/adults, toxic substances for recreational purposes or overdose taken with intent to produce self-harm

    c. Epidemiology

        1) Nearly 50% of cases occur in children <6 yr old, as a result of an accidental event or as abuse

        2) Ninety-two percent occur at home, 60% with nonpharmacologic agent, 40% with pharmacologic agent

        3) Ingestion occurs in 75% of cases, 8% dermal, 6% ophthalmic, 6% inhalation

    d. Hx is crucial during initial contact with patient or guardian

        1) Evaluation of severity (asymptomatic, symptomatic)

        2) Age & weight

        3) Time, type, amount, & route of exposure

        4) Past medical history

    e. Si/Sx (Table 6)

    f. Tx

        1) Syrup of ipecac followed by clear liquid (water) induces vomiting, should not use in children <6 mo, those with depressed sensorium, those with seizures, or who ingested strong acids or bases

        2) Lavage usually unnecessary in children, may be useful with drugs that decrease gastric motility

        3) Charcoal may be most effective & safest procedure to prevent absorption, repeat doses every 2–6 hr with cathartic for first dose, ineffective in heavy metal or volatile hydrocarbon poisoning

TABLE 6	Pediatric Toxicology
SI/SX	**POSSIBLE TOXIN**
Lethargy/Coma	Ethanol, sedative-hypnotics, narcotics, antihistamines, antidepressants, neuroleptic
Seizures	Theophylline, cocaine, amphetamines, antidepressants, antipsychotics, pesticides
Hypotension (with bradycardia)	Organophosphate pesticides, beta blockers
Arrhythmia	Tricyclic antidepressants, cocaine, digitalis, quinidine
Hyperthermia	Salicylates, anticholinergics
Drooling, severe pain in mouth, abdomen, chest	Lye (alkali agents)

B. Adolescence

1. Epidemiology

   a. Injuries

      1) Fifty percent of all deaths in adolescents attributed to injuries

      2) Many occur under the influence of alcohol & other drugs

      3) Older adolescents more likely to be killed in motor vehicle accidents, while younger adolescents are at risk for drowning & fatal injuries with weapons

      4) Homicide rate is 5× higher for black males than white males

   b. Suicide

      1) Second leading cause of adolescent death

      2) Females more likely to attempt than males, but males are 5× more likely to succeed than females

      3) Pts with preexisting psychiatric problems or those who abuse alcohol & drugs more likely to attempt suicide

   c. Substance abuse

      1) A major cause of morbidity in adolescents

      2) Average age of first use is 12–14 yr old

      3) One of every two adolescents have tried an illicit drug by their high school graduation

      4) Survey of high school seniors (1994–1995) noted that 90% had experience with alcohol & ≥40% had tried marijuana

  d. Sex

      1) Sixty-one percent of all male & 47% of all female high school students have had sex

      2) Health risks of early sexual activity are unwanted pregnancies and sexually transmitted diseases (STDs) such as gonorrhea, *Chlamydia,* & HIV

      3) Eighty-six percent of all STDs occur among adolescents & young adults 15–29 yr old

      4) More than 1 million adolescent females become pregnant yearly, 33% are <15 yr old—this is a second major cause of morbidity in adolescents

2. Confidentiality

  a. Most issues revealed by adolescents to physicians in an interview are confidential

  b. **Exceptions** include suicidal or homicidal behavior, sexual or physical abuse

  c. It is strongly encouraged that physicians inform adolescents about confidentiality at the beginning of the interview to help develop a trusting relationship between adolescent & physician

V. CHILD AND ADOLESCENT PSYCHIATRY

A. Autism & Asperger's Syndrome

1. Autism is the prototypic **pervasive developmental disorder**, pervasive because the disorder encompasses so many areas of development: language, social interaction, and emotional reactivity

2. The expression "living in his own world" captures this tragic disorder; the autistic child fails to develop normal interactions with others & seems to be responding to internal stimuli

3. Si/Sx

  a. Becomes evident before 3 years of age, often much earlier

    b. The baby does not seem to be concerned with the mother's presence or absence & makes no eye contact, as the baby becomes older, deficiencies in language (including repetitive phrases & made-up vocabulary), & abnormal behavior become more obvious

    c. Look for the behavioral aspects; the child often has a strange, persistent fascination with specific, seemingly mundane objects (vacuum cleaners, sprinklers) & may show stereotyped, ritualistic movements (e.g., spinning around)

    d. Autistic children have an inordinate need for constancy

4. Think of Asperger's syndrome as autism **without** the language impairment

5. **Contrary to previous thought, poor parenting/bonding is not a cause of autism! Parents need reassurance about this**

6. The treatment for Autism & Aspergers is psychosocial support for the patient and family

B. Depression

1. Depression may present slightly differently depending on the age group

    a. Preschool children may be hyperactive & aggressive

    b. Adolescents show boredom, irritability, or openly antisocial behaviors

2. One should still look for the same symptoms as described for adult depression: depressed mood, anhedonia, neurovegetative changes, etc.

3. Tx

    a. Unlike adult depression, the use of antidepressants is much more controversial, with far less data supporting its effectiveness

    b. **Note:** Children's mood disorders are especially sensitive to psychosocial stressors, so family therapy is a major consideration

C. Separation Anxiety

1. Look for a child that seems a bit too attached to his parents or any other figures in his life; the child is worried that something will happen to these beloved figures or that some terrible event will separate them

2. Si/Sx = sleep disturbances (nightmares, inability to fall asleep alone) & somatic Sx during times of separation (headaches, stomach upset at school)

3. Tx = desensitizing therapy (gradually increasing the hours spent away from Mom & Dad), in some cases imipramine is used

D. Oppositional Defiant/Conduct Disorder

1. Differentiate the two by words & action

2. Oppositional defiant disorder Si/Sx ("bark")

   a. Pts are argumentative, temperamental, & defiant, more so with people they know well (they may seem harmless to you)

   b. Big surprise that they are often friendless & perform poorly in school

3. Conduct disorder Si/Sx ("bite")

   a. Pts bully others, start fights, may show physical cruelty to animals, violate/destroy other people's property (fire-setting), steal things, & stay out past curfews or run away

   b. They do not feel guilty for any of this

   c. A glimpse into the child's family life often reveals pathology in the form of substance abuse or negligence

4. Oppositional defiant disorder may lead to conduct disorder, but the two are not synonymous

5. Tx = providing a setting with strict rules & expected consequences for violations of them

E. Attention-Deficit Hyperactivity Disorder (ADHD)

1. Si/Sx can be divided into the components suggested by their name

   a. Attention-deficit Sx = inability to focus or carry out tasks completely, and easily distracted by random stimuli

   b. Hyperactivity Sx are more outwardly motor; the child is unable to sit still, talks excessively, & can never "wait his turn" in group games

2. Dx requires that Sx have been present since before 7 years of age

3. Tx = methylphenidate, an amphetamine

a. Parents & teachers notice improvement in the child's behavior

b. Because of concerns about impeding the child's growth, drug holidays are often taken (e.g., no meds over weekends or vacations)

c. Children with ADHD also do better with an extremely structured environment featuring consistent rules & punishments

d. Px is variable, some children show remissions of their hyperactivity, but quite a few continue to show Sx through adolescence & adulthood; children with ADHD have a higher likelihood of developing conduct disorders or antisocial personalities

F. Tourette's Disorder

1. Tics are involuntary, stereotyped, repetitive movements or vocalizations

2. **Tourette's Dx requires both a motor tic & a vocal tic present for ≥1 yr**

3. **The vocal tics are often obscene or socially unacceptable (copralalia)**, which is a cause of extreme embarrassment to the patient

4. Tx = haloperidol, effective, but not required in mild cases

5. Psychotherapy is unhelpful in treating the tics per se, but can be helpful in dealing with the emotional stress caused by the disorder

G. Anorexia & Bulimia Nervosa

1. Eating disorders are by no means limited to children—but because they often start in adolescence, they are worth mentioning here

2. In both disorders exists a profound disturbance in body image & its role in the person's sense of self-worth

3. Anorexia

a. Anorexia nervosa occurs in 0.5% of adolescent females. Two peak ages are 14.5 yr and 18 yr, but 25% may be <13 yr old

b. **By definition, anorexic patients are below their expected body weight** because they do not eat enough, often creating elaborate rituals for disposing of food in meal settings, e.g., cutting meat into tiny pieces and rearranging them constantly on the plate

   c. **Amenorrhea occurs 2° to weight loss,** also see constipation

4. Bulimia

   a. Occurs in 1–3% of adolescent females

   b. More common than anorexia, **characterized by binge eating**: consuming huge amounts of food over a short period, with a perceived lack of control

   c. This may be accompanied by active purging (vomiting, laxative use)

   d. **Unlike anorexics, who by definition have decreased body weight, bulemics often have a normal appearance**

   e. **Abrasions over the knuckles** (from jamming the fingers into the mouth to induce vomiting), **dental erosion,** parotid gland enlargement, and tooth decay are all classic findings

5. Tx

   a. Hospitalization may be required for anorexia to restore the pt's weight to a safe level, which the pt will often resist

   b. Because of vomiting, monitoring serum electrolytes is essential; the most worrisome consequence is cardiac dysfunction—as exemplified by singer Karen Carpenter, whose battle with anorexia led to her untimely death

   c. Psychotherapy is the mainstay of Tx for both diseases

6. Overall, anorexia nervosa has a relatively poor prognosis, with persistent preoccupations with food & weight; bulimics fare slightly better

VI. DRUGS OF ABUSE

1. Always consider drug abuse when a pt's life seems to be going down the tubes, e.g., deteriorating family relations, work performance, financial stability

2. Generally (with many exceptions) withdrawal Sx are the opposite of intoxication; dysphoria is characteristic of all of them—**withdrawal is a sign of physiologic dependence**

3. Individual drugs (Table 7)

TABLE 7	Drug Intoxications and Withdrawal	
DRUG	**INTOXICATION SI/SX**	**WITHDRAWAL**
Alcohol	Disinhibition, ↓ cognition screen for alcoholism with CAGE • C—feeling the need to **cut** down • A—feeling **annoyed** when asked about drinking • G—feeling **guilty** for drinking • E—need a drink in the morning **(eye-opener)**	Tremor, seizures, delirium tremens (high mortality! → prevent with benzo's)
Cocaine/ amphetamine	Agitation, irritability, ↓ appetite, formication, ↑ or ↓ BP & HR, cardiac arrhythmia or infarction, stroke, seizure, nosebleeds	Hypersomnolence, dysphoria ↑ appetite
Heroin (opioids)	Intense, fleeting euphoria, drowsy, slurred speech, ↓ memory, pupillary constriction, ↓ respiration **The triad of ↓ consciousness, pinpoint pupils & respiratory depression should always lead to a suspicion of opioids**	Nausea/vomiting, pupillary dilation & insomnia
Benzodiazepine & barbiturates	Respiratory & cardiac depression	Agitation, anxiety, delirium
Phencyclidine (PCP)	Intense psychosis, violence, rhabdomyolysis, hyperthermia	
LSD	Sensation is enhanced, colors are richer, music more profound, tastes heightened	

VII. PSYCHIATRY/MOOD DISORDERS

A. DSM-IV (Diagnostic & Statistical Manual)

1. The DSM-IV lists current US diagnostic criteria for psychiatric conditions
2. **The USMLE will rely on DSM-IV diagnostic criteria**
3. **Do not try memorizing all the possible Sx mentioned by the DSM** to define a given condition. It is impossible and not a good use of time. This review will focus on the Sx you are **most likely to see on the exam**
4. DSM IV Classification (Table 8)

TABLE 8	DSM-IV Classification
AXIS I	Clinical disorders
AXIS II	Personality disorders/mental retardation
AXIS III	Medical conditions
AXIS IV	Social and environmental factors
AXIS V	Level of functioning

B. Principles of Psychiatry for the USMLE (More Complex in Real Life)

1. Major psychiatric dx requires **significant impairment in the pt's life**
2. **Always rule out drug abuse** (frequent comorbidity in psychiatric dz)
3. **Combination Tx** (pharmacology & psychotherapy) **is superior** to either alone but **pharmacologic Tx is first line for severe dz in acute setting**
4. **Criteria for hospitalization (any single criterion is acceptable)**
   a. Danger to self (suicide)
   b. Danger to others
   c. Unable to provide food, clothing, shelter (grave disability)
5. Psychiatric dz is chronic—if asked about dz course, **"cures" are rare**
6. Prognosis depends on symptom onset, insight & premorbid function
7. Prognosis of Psychiatric Disorders (Table 9)

TABLE 9	Prognosis of Psychiatric Disorders		
PROGNOSIS	**SYMPTOM ONSET**	**INSIGHT***	**PREMORBID FUNCTION**
Favorable	Acute	Good	High
Unfavorable	Subacute/chronic	Poor	Low
* Insight = pt recognizes symptoms as abormalities & is distressed by them.			

C. Mood Disorders (Table 10)

TABLE 10	Mood Disorders
DISORDER	**Si/Sx**
Major Depressive Disorder (MDD)	Two depressive episodes of 2 weeks duration, 2 months apart; ↓ mood, anhedonia, insomnia, ↓ appetite, weight loss, fatigue, ↓ concentration, guilt or feeling worthless, recurrent thoughts of death & suicide
Dysthymic Disorder	Continuous depressive symptoms for a minimum of 2 yr. Dysthymic disorder is longer but less acute than MDD
Bereavement	Depressive symptoms occuring soon after a death. If Sxs persist for >2 mo, Dx is MDD rather than normal bereavement
Bipolar Disorder (Manic-Depression)	Often presents in young people, while major depression is a dz of middle age (40s). Abrupt onset of ↑ energy, ↓ need to sleep, pressured speech (speaks quickly to the point of making no sense), ↓ attention span, hypersexuality, spending large amounts of money, engaging in outrageous activities. Episodes **must last ≥1 wk & should be abrupt, not continuous** **Hypomania = Presents with identical Sxs of mania but manic episodes cause significant disability** while hypomania doesn't. **Bipolar I** = manic episode with or without depressive episodes (pts often have depressive episodes before experiencing mania) **Bipolar II** = depressive episodes **with hypomanic episodes**, but by definition, **the absence of manic episodes** **Rapid cycling** = four episodes (depressive, manic, or mixed) in 12 mo; can be precipitated by antidepressants
Drug-Induced Mania	Cocaine & amphetamines are major culprits. Tachycardia, hypertension, dilated pupils, **EKG arrhythmia or ischemia in young people is highly suggestive** Urine or serum toxicology screen diagnostic

D. Treatment

1. **Depression**

   a. Psychotherapy = psychodynamic (understanding self/inner conflicts), cognitive-behavioral (recognizing negative thought or behavior & altering thinking/behavior accordingly), interpersonal (examines relation of Sx to negative/absent relationships with others)

TABLE 11	Pharmacologic Therapy for Depression[a]	
DRUG	**EXAMPLES**	**SIDE EFFECTS**
SSRIs[b]	Fluoxetine, paroxetine	Favorable profile: rare impotence
TCAs[b]	Amitriptyline, desipramine, imipramine, nortriptyline	More severe: confusion, sedation, **orthostatic hypotension, prolonged QRS duration** (think autonomic/cholinergic)
MAO[b] Inhibitors	Phenelzine, tranylcypromine	Very severe: classic syndromes • **Serotonin syndrome** = caused by **MAO inhibitor interaction with SSRIs, demerol, or pseudoephedrine** & others, presents with hyperthermia, muscle rigidity, altered mental status • **Hypertensive crisis** = malignant hypertension when ingested with foods rich in **tyramine** (wine & cheese)

[a]Takes 2–6 wk for effect.
[b]SSRIs (selective serotonin reuptake inhibitors) are first line; TCAs (tricyclic antidepressants) are second line; MAO inhibitors (monoamine oxidase inhibitors) are third line.

    b. Electroconvulsive therapy (ECT) is effective for refractory cases, main side effect is short-term memory loss

    c. Pharmacologic Therapy for Depression (Table 11)

2. **Mania**

    a. Hospitalization, often involuntary since manic pts rarely see the need

    b. **Valproate** or **carbamazepine** are first line, **lithium** second line

    c. Valproate and carbamazepine cause **blood dyscrasias**

    d. Lithium blood levels must be checked due to frequent toxicity, including **tremor** and polyuria due to **nephrogenic diabetes insipidus**

    e. Px worse than major depression, episodes more frequent with age

    f. Calcium-channel blockers used in drug-induced mania for acute autonomic Sxs, drug Tx programs longer term

VIII. PSYCHOSIS

A. Hallucinations & Delusions are Hallmark

1. Hallucination = false sensory perception not based on real stimulus
2. Delusion = false interpretation of external reality. Can be paranoid, grandiose (thinking one possesses special powers), religious (God is talking to the pt), or ideas of reference (every event in the world somehow involves the pt)

B. DDx (Table 12)

TABLE 12	Diagnosis of Psychotic Disorders
DISEASE	**CHARACTERISTICS**
Schizophrenia	• **Presents in late teens—20s (slightly later in women), very strong genetic predisposition** • Often accompanied by **premorbid** signs, including poor school performance, poor emotional expression & lack of friends • Positive Sx = hallucinations (**more often auditory than visual**) & delusions • Negative Sx = lack of affect, alogia • Other Sx = disorganized behavior &/or speech • **Schizophrenia lasts ≥6 mo continuously** • **Schizophreniform disorder lasts 1–6 mo** • **Brief psychotic disorder lasts 1 day–1 mo**, with full recovery of baseline functioning—look for acute stressor, e.g., the death of a loved one
Other Psychoses	• Schizoaffective disorder = meets criteria for mood disorders & schizophrenia • Delusional disorder = **nonbizarre delusions** (they could happen, e.g., pt's spouse is unfaithful, a person who is trying to kill the pt, etc.), without hallucinations, disorganized speech or disorganized behavior
Mood disorders	• Major depression & bipolar disorder can cause delusions & in extreme cases, hallucination can be difficult to differentiate from schizophrenia
Delirium	• Seen in pts with underlying illnesses, often in ICU (ICU psychosis) • **Patients are not orientated to person, place, time** • **Severity waxes & wanes even during the course of 1 day** • Resolves with treatment of underlying dz
Drugs	• LSD & PCP → predominantly visual, taste, touch, or olfactory hallucination • Cocaine & amphetamines → paranoid delusions & **classic sensation of bugs crawling on the skin (formication)** • Anabolic steroids → body-builder with bad temper, acne, shrunken testicles • Corticosteroids → psychosis/mood disturbances early in course of therapy
Medical	• Metabolic, endocrine, neoplastic & seizure dz can all cause psychosis • **Look for associated Si/Sx not explained by psychosis**, including focal neurologic findings, seizure, sensory/motor deficits, abnormal lab values

C. Tx

1. Hospitalization: to protect patient from hurting self or others, or if condition is disabling to the point that pts cannot care for themselves
2. Pharmacologic therapy
   a. Dopamine-blockers mainstay of treatment
   b. Differences among agents relate to side-effect profile
   c. Compliance to drugs can be improved with **depot** form of haloperidol, which administers a month's supply of drug in 1 IM injection
3. Psychotherapy can improve social functioning
   a. Behavioral: social skills that allow pts to deal more comfortably with other people
   b. Family-oriented: help family members to act in more appropriate, positive fashion
4. Antipsychotic Drugs (Table 13)

TABLE 13	Antipsychotic Drugs	
DRUG		**ADVERSE EFFECTS**[a]
		Typical Antipsychotics[b]
Chlorpromazine	Low potency	↑ anticholinergic effects, ↓ movement disorders
Haloperidol	High potency	↓ anticholinergic effects, ↑ movement disorders
		Atypical Antipsychotics[b]
Clozapine	For refractory dz	1% incidence of agranulocytosis mandates weekly CBC
Risperidone	First line	Minimal
Olanzapine	First line	Minimal

[a]Anticholinergic effects = dry mouth, blurry vision (miosis), urinary retention, constipation.
[b]Atypical agents have much lower incidence of movement disorders—see Table 14.

TABLE 14	Antipsychotic Associated Movements Disorders	
DISORDER	**TIME COURSE**	**CHARACTERISTICS**
Acute dystonia	4 hr → 4 days	• Sustained muscle spasm anywhere in the body but often in neck (torticollis), jaw, or back (opisthotonos) • Tx = immediate IV diphenhydramine
Parkinsonism	4 days → 4 mo	• Cog-wheel rigidity, shuffling gait, resting tremor • Tx = benztropine (anticholinergic)
Tardive dyskinesia	4 mo → 4 yr	• Involuntary, irregular movements of the head, tongue, lips, limbs & trunk • Tx = immediately change medication or ↓ doses because effects are often permanent
Akathisia	Any time	• Subjective sense of discomfort → restlessness: pacing, sitting down & getting up • Tx = lower medication doses
Neuroleptic malignant syndrome	Any time	• Life-threatening muscle rigidity → fever, ↑ BP/HR, rhabdomyolysis appearing over 1–3 days • Can be easily misdiagnosed as ↑ psychotic Sx • Labs →↑ WBC, ↑ creatine kinase, ↑ transaminases, ↑ plasma myoglobin, as well as myoglobinuria • Tx = supportive: immediately stop drug, give dantrolene (inhibits Ca release into cells), cool pt to prevent hyperpyrexia

5. Antipsychotic Associated Movements (Table 14)

D. Px

1. Schizophrenia is a chronic, episodic dz, recovery from each relapse typically leaves pt below former baseline function

2. Presence of negative Sx (e.g., flat affect) marks poor Px

3. High-functioning prior to psychotic break marks better Px

IX. ANXIETY DISORDERS

TABLE 15	Anxiety Disorders	
DIAGNOSIS	SI/SXs	TREATMENT
Panic Disorder	Mimics MI: chest pain, palpitations, diaphoresis, nausea, marked anxiety, escalate for 10 min, remain for about 30 min; occurs in younger pts (average age 25); panic attacks are unexpected, unlike phobias which consistently occur in certain settings. Diagnosis of exclusion	TCAs (clomipramine & imipramine) are best studied. More recently SSRIs have been shown to have longer efficacy. Benzodiazepenes work immediately, have ↑ risk of addiction. Therefore, start benzodiazepenes for immediate effects, add a TCA or SSRI, taper off the benzodiazepenes as the other drugs kick in Cognitive/behavior TX & respiratory training (to help patients recognize & overcome desire to hyperventilate) are helpful
Agoraphobia	Fear of being in situations where it would be very difficult to get out should a panic attack arise. Evidence of social/occupational dysfunction	β-blockers useful for prophylaxis in phobias related to performance Exposure desensitization = exposure to noxious stimulus in increments, while undergoing concurrent relaxation Tx
Obsessive Compulsive Disorder (OCD)	Obsessive thought causes anxiety & the compulsion is a way of temporarily relieving that anxiety. Obsessions commonly involve: cleanliness/contamination (washing hands), doubt, symmetry (elaborate rituals for entering doorways, arranging books, etc.) & sex. Pt should be disturbed by their obsessions & should recognize their absurdity in contrast to obsessive compulsive personality disorder, where pt sees nothing wrong with compulsion	SSRIs (first line) or clomipramine, psychotherapy in which the pt is literally forced to overcome their behavior

TABLE 15	*Continued*	
DIAGNOSIS	**SI/SXs**	**TREATMENT**
Posttraumatic Stress Disorder (PTSD)	Requires a traumatic, violent incident that effectively scars the person involved; the experiences of Vietnam vets are emblematic of this disorder **Pt relives the initial incident via conscious thoughts or dreams** Due to resultant subjective & physiologic distress, the pt avoids any precipitating stimuli & **hence often avoids public places & activities** Pt may suffer restricted emotional involvement/responses & may experience a detachment from others **Depression is common, look for moodiness, diminished interest in activities & difficulties with sleeping & concentrating**	Use of tricyclics (imipramine & amitriptyline) is well-supported by clinical trials, SSRIs have also been used. **Beware of giving benzodiazepenes due to a high association of substance abuse with PTSD!** Psychotherapy takes two approaches Exposure therapy, the idea being to confront one's demons by "reliving" the experience Relaxation techniques, think of the two modalities as attacking the source vs. controlling the symptoms
Generalized Anxiety Disorder	Worry most days for at least 6 mo, irritability, inability to concentrate, insomnia, fatigue, restlessness **Dx requires evidence of social dysfunction** (e.g., poor school grades, job stagnation, or marital strains) to rule out "normal" anxiety	Psychotherapy due to chronicity of the problem a. Cognitive-behavioral Tx teaching pt to recognize his/her worrying & find ways to respond to it through behavior & thought patterns b. **Biofeedback & relaxation** techniques, in particular, can help the pt deal with physical manifestations of anxiety, e.g., heart rate c. Pharmacotherapy includes buspirone or β-blockers

X. PERSONALITY DISORDERS

A. General Characteristics

1. Sx = pervasive pattern of maladaptive behavior causing functional impairment, consistent behavior can often be traced back to childhood

2. Typically present to psychiatrists because behavior is causing significant problems for others, e.g., colleagues at work, spouse at home, **or for the medical staff in the inpatient or clinic setting (typical USMLE question)**

3. **Pts usually see nothing wrong with their behavior (ego-syntonic)**, contrast with pts who recognize their hallucinations as abnormal (ego-dystonic)

4. Ego defenses

   a. Unconscious mental process that individuals resort to in order to quell inner conflicts & anxiety that are unacceptable to the ego

   b. Examples include "splitting" & "projection"

5. Tx = psychotherapy, medication used for peripheral Sx (e.g., anxiety)

B. Clusters

1. **Cluster A** = paranoid, schizoid & schizotypal personalities, often thought of as **"weird" or "eccentric"**

2. **Cluster B** = borderline, antisocial, histrionic, & narcissistic personalities, **"dramatic"** & **"aggressive"** personalities

3. **Cluster C** = avoidant, dependent, & obsessive-compulsive personalities, **"shy"** & **"nervous"** personalities

C. Specific Personality Disorders (Table 16)

TABLE 16	Specific Personality Disorders
DISORDER	**CHARACTERISTICS**
Paranoid (Cluster A)	• Negatively misinterpret the actions, words, intentions of others • Often utilize **projection** as ego defense (attributing to other people impulses & thoughts that are unacceptable to their own selves) • **Do not hold fixed delusions** (delusional disorder), **nor do they experience hallucinations** (schizophrenia)
Schizoid (Cluster A)	• Socially withdrawn, introverted, with little external affect • Do not form close emotional ties with others (often feel no need) • Are, however, able to recognize reality
Schizotypal (Cluster A)	• **Believe in concepts not considered real by the rest of society (magic, clairvoyance),** display the prototypal ego defense: **fantasy** • Not necessarily psychotic (can have brief psychotic episodes) • Like schizoids, they are often quite isolated socially • **Often related to schizophrenics (unlike other cluster A disorders)**
Antisocial (Cluster B)	• Violate the rights of others, break the law (e.g., theft, substance abuse) • Can also be quite seductive (particularly with the opposite sex) • **For Dx the pt must have exhibited the behavior by a certain age (15—think truancy) but must be a certain age (at least 18—adult)** • **A popular USMLE topic; you may have to differentiate it from conduct disorder (bad behavior, but Dx of children/adolescents)**
Borderline (Cluster B)	• Volatile emotional lives, swing wildly between idealizing & devaluing other people: (**splitting** ego defense = people are very good or bad) • **Also commonly asked on USMLE**, typical scenario is a highly disruptive hospitalized pt; on interview, he (but usually she) says some nurses are incompetent & cruel but wildly praises others (including you) • Exhibit self-destructive behavior (scratching or cutting themselves) • Ability to **disassociate**: they simply "forget" negative affects/experiences by covering them with overly exuberant, seemingly positive behavior
Histrionic (Cluster B)	• Require the attention of everyone, use sexuality & physical appearance to get it, exaggerate their thoughts with dramatic but vague language Utilize disassociation & **repression** (block feelings unconsciously)—don't confuse with **suppression** (feelings put aside consciously)

TABLE 16	*Continued*
DISORDER	**CHARACTERISTICS**
Narcissistic (Cluster B)	• Feel entitled—strikingly so—because they are the best & everyone else is inferior, handle criticism very poorly
Dependent (Cluster C)	• Can do little on their own, nor can they be alone
Avoidant (Cluster C)	• Feel inadequate & are extremely sensitive to negative comments • Reluctant to try new things (e.g., making friends) for fear of embarrassment
Obsessive-compulsive (Cluster C)	• Preoccupied with detail: rules, regulations, neatness • Isolation is a common ego-defense: putting up walls of self-restraint & detail-orientation that keep away any sign of emotional affect

D. Other Ego Defenses

1. Acting out = transforming unacceptable feeling into actions, often loud ones (tantrums)
2. Identification = patterning behavior after someone else's
3. Intellectualization = explaining away the unreasonable in the form of logic
4. Rationalization = making the unreasonable seem acceptable (e.g., upon being fired, you say you wanted to quit anyway)
5. Reaction formation = set aside unconscious feelings & express exactly opposite feelings (show extra affection for someone you hate)
6. Regression = resorting to childlike behavior (often seen in the hospital)
7. Sublimation = taking instinctual drives (sex) & funneling that energy into a socially acceptable action (studying)

XI. SOMATOFORM AND FACTITIOUS DISORDERS

A. Definitions

1. Somatoform disorder = **lack of conscious manipulation of somatic Sx**

2. Factitious disorder = **consciously faking** or manipulating Sx for purpose of "assuming the sick role," **but not for material gain**

3. Malingering = consciously faking Sx **for purpose of material gain**

B. Factitious Disorder

1. Pt may mimic any Sx, physical or psychological, to assume the sick role

2. **The patient is not trying to avoid work or win a compensation claim**

3. Munchausen syndrome = factitious disorder with predominantly physical (not psychological) symptoms

4. Munchausen by proxy = pt claiming nonexistent symptoms in someone else under their care, e.g., parents bringing in their "sick" children

5. DDx = malingering

6. **HINT: the USMLE will very likely present a scenario involving nurses or other health care workers as the pts (often involving an episode of apparent hypoglycemia), look for evidence of factitious disorder (e.g., low C-peptide levels suggesting insulin self-injection)**

7. Dx is by exclusion of real medical condition

8. Tx is nearly impossible; when confronted, pts often become angry, deny everything, tell you how horrible you are & move on to someone else

C. Somatoform Disorders

1. Somatization disorder

   a. Often female pts with problems starting before age 30, with history of frequent visits to the doctor for countless procedures & operations (often exploratory), & often history of abusive/failed relationships

   b. Sx = somatic complaints involving different systems, particularly gastrointestinal (nausea, diarrhea), neurologic (weakness), & sexual (irregular menses), with no adequate medical explanation on the basis of exam/lab findings

   c. Dx = rule out medical condition & material or psychologic
gain

   d. Tx = **continuity of care**

   1) Schedule regular appointments so pt can express his or
her Sx

   2) Perform physical exam but do not order laboratory tests

   3) As the therapeutic bond strengthens, strive to establish
awareness in the pt that psychologic factors are
involved & if successful in doing so, arrange a psychiatric consult, but if done too early or aggressively, pt
may be reluctant or resentful

2. Conversion disorder

   a. Sx are neurologic, not multisystem, & are not consciously faked

   b. Sensory deficits often fail to correspond to any known
pathway, e.g., a stocking-&-glove sensory deficit that
begins precisely at the wrist, studies will reveal intact
neurologic pathways, & pts rarely get hurt, e.g., patients
who are "blind" will not be colliding into the wall

   c. Dx requires identification of a stressor that precipitated
the Sx, as well as exclusion of any adequate medical explanation (**NOTE:** in some studies 50% of pts who received
this Dx were eventually found to have nonpsychiatric
causes of illness, e.g., brain tumors & multiple sclerosis.
Bummer!)

   d. Tx = supportive, Sx resolve within days (less than a month),
**do not tell pt that they are imagining their Sx, but sug-
gest that psychotherapy may help with their distress**

   e. Px = the more abrupt the symptoms, the more easily iden-
tified the stressor; & the higher the premorbid function,
the better the outcome

3. Hypochondriasis

   a. Sx = preoccupation with disease, pt does not complain of
a large number of Sx but misinterprets them as evidence
of something serious

   b. Tx = regular visits to MD with every effort not to order lab
tests or procedures, psychotherapy should be presented as
a way of coping with stress, **again, do not tell patients
that they are imagining their Sx**

4. Body dysmorphic disorder

a. Sx = concern with body, **pt usually picks one feature, often on the face, & imagines deficits that other people do not see;** if there are slight imperfections, the pt exaggerates them excessively

b. Look for a significant amount of emotional & functional impairment

c. Tx = SSRIs may be helpful in some cases, surgery is not recommended

XII. MISCELLANEOUS DISORDERS

A. Disorders of Sexuality & Gender Identity

1. Sexual identity is based on biology, e.g., men have testes

2. Gender identity is based on self-perception, e.g., biological male perceives himself as a male

3. **Children have a firm conception of their gender identity very early (before age 3)**

4. Sexual orientation is who the person is attracted to; **remember that homosexuality is not a psychiatric disorder** (it used to be, until taken off the DSM in the 1970s) & that treating crises of sexual orientation should focus on accepting one's orientation, not changing it to conform to social "norms"

B. Disassociative Disorder (Multiple Personality Disorder)

1. This was a hot diagnosis in the late 1970s (replaced in 1980s by borderline personality) & a perennial favorite of the movies (think: *Three Faces of Eve, Sybil,* & more recently, *Primal Fear*). The older name says it all: a patient seemingly possesses different personalities that can each take control at a given time. A patient's history may indicate childhood trauma, e.g., abuse. Treatment focuses on gradual integration of these personalities

2. The main differentials are **dissociative amnesia & dissociative fugue.** Amnesia is a syndrome of forgetting a great deal of personal information; fugue refers to the syndrome of sudden travel to another place, with inability to remember the past & confusion of present identity. *Neither case involves shifting between different identities*

C. Adjustment Disorder

1. This refers to any behavioral or emotional Sx that occur in response to stressful life events in excess of what is normal

2. Obviously has a catch-all quality to it; **this will be a frequent answer option on the USMLE**

3. **Dx requires the Sx to come within 3 mo of the stressor** (so they do not have to be immediate) & **they must disappear within 6 mo of the disappearance of the stressor**

4. Bereavement may seem to be a type of adjustment disorder (the stressor being death), but they are separate diagnoses

5. Depending on the setting, adjustment disorder may appear as depression or anxiety—so how to tell the difference? It isn't easy, but remember: **axis I disorders such as major depression & generalized anxiety take precedence**

D. Impulsive-Control Disorders

1. Pt is unable to resist the drive to perform certain actions **harmful to themselves or others**

2. Note the emotional response: these individuals **feel anxiety before the action & gratification afterward**

3. *Intermittent explosive disorder*

   a. Discrete episodes of aggressive behavior far in excess of any possible stressor

   b. The key term is **episodic**; antisocial personalities also commit aggressive behaviors, but their aggression is present between outbursts of such behavior

4. *Kleptomania*: the impulse to steal

   a. The object of theft is not needed for any reason (monetary or otherwise)

   b. The kleptomaniac often feels guilty after stealing

5. *Pyromania*: purposeful fire-setting

   a. There is often a fascination with fire itself that distinguishes this from the antisocial personality/conduct disorders, where the fire-setting is purposeful, e.g., revenge, & not the failure to resist an impulse

7. *Trichotillomania*: hair-pulling, resulting in observable hair loss

TABLE 17	Dementia versus Delirium	
	DEMENTIA	**DELIRIUM**
Definition	Both cause global decline in cognition, memory, personality, motor, or sensory functions	
Course	Constant, progressive	Sudden onset, waxing/waning daily
Reversible?	Usually not	Almost always
Circadian?	Constant, no daily pattern	Usually worse at night (sun-downing)
Consciousness	Normal	Altered (obtunded)
Hallucination	Usually not	Often, classically visual
Tremor	Often not	Often present (i.e., asterixis)
Causes	Alzheimer's, multi-infarct, Pick's dz, alcohol, brain infxn/tumors, malnutrition (thiamine/B_{12} deficiency)	Systemic infection/neoplasm, drugs (**particularly narcotics & benzodiazepines**), stroke, heart dz, alcoholism, uremia, electrolyte imbalance, hyper/hypoglycemia
Treatment	Supportive—see below for specifics depending on the disease	Treat underlying cause, **control Sx with haloperidol instead of sedatives**—due to agitation pts are often given benzodiazepines or sedatives, but these drugs often exacerbate the delirium as they disorient the pt even more

XIII. SLEEP

A. Normal Sleep

    1. There are two different types of sleep

        a. Non rapid eye movement (NREM)

            1) Four stages (see Table 18)

        b. Rapid eye movement (REM)

B. Sleep Stages (Table 18)

TABLE 18	Sleep Stages
STAGES	**CHARACTERISTICS**
Non-REM	Early slow wave sleep
Stage 1	Alpha waves (Awake waves disappear) and Theta waves (Time to sleep waves occur)
Stage 2	Sleep spindles
Stages 3 & 4	Delta wave sleep (most difficult to awake from)
REM	Dreaming (suppressed by alcohol and drugs)

C. Sleep Disorders

1. Dysnomnias: Difficulties with Sleep

    a. Insomnia

    1) Unable to fall asleep or stay asleep recurrently over a month's time

    2) Can be associated with stress, anxiety, drugs, and various medical and mental conditions

    3) Tx-sleep routine, exercise, antihistamines, short course of benzodiazepenes <2 wk to prevent rebound insomnia

    b. Hypersomnia

    1) Narcolepsy-recurrent sleep attacks, associated with REM sleep and dreaming

        a) Pts can suddenly collapse due to loss of all muscle tone (Cataplexy)

        b) Tx-stimulants such as methylphenidate or pemoline

    2) Sleep apnea: periods of apnea occurring during sleep

        a) Obstructive-increased inspiratory effort that fails to result in increased airflow

            i) Most common, patients are usually obese heavy snorers who awake after a gasp for air. Pts complain of excessive daytime sleepiness. Spouse complains of loud snoring

            ii) Can lead to pulmonary hypertension, associated with hypothyroidism

            iii) Tx-weight loss, continuos positive airway pressure (CPAP) at night to maintain patent airway.

Surgery if no relief and severely affecting lifestyle or danger to life.

   b) Mixed obstructive/central: Periods of no inspiratory effort followed by inspiratory effort that is obstructed by collapse of oropharyngeal airway

   c) Central sleep apnea: rare, loss of inspiratory effort

3) Pickwickian syndrome (central alveolar hypoventilation)

   a) Triad of somnolence, obesity, and erythrocytosis

   b) Gradual onset of hypercapnea, hypoxemia, and erythrocytosis

   c) Weight of adipose tissue on lungs and abdomen cause a chronic alveolar hypoventilation

   d) Tx-weight loss

2. Parasomnias

  a. Night terror

   1) Arises during NREM sleep

   2) Child sits up suddenly in bed with diaphoresis, tachycardia, and frightened

   3) Not fully awake, patients usually fall back to sleep after the episode

  b. Nightmares

   1) Occur during REM sleep

   2) Usually after an emotional event, stress, or frightening movie

   3) Patients are fully awake, have good recall of nightmare events

   4) Also associated with drugs

  c. Sleep walking (somnambulism)

   1) Occurs during NREM sleep

   2) Patients get out of bed and wander around, some patients can jump out of windows or open doors

   3) Patients usually awaken with no memory of events

XIV. NUTRITION

A. Nutritional Assessment

1. Diet history: Many methods can be used to assess a patients nutritional status. Whatever method used must start with a careful history of nutritional intake

2. Laboratory studies occasionally used;

   a. Serum albumin levels: Half life 18–20 days, normal levels 3.5–5.5 g/dL, severe malnutrition <2.1 g/dL

   b. Serum prealbumin levels: Half life 2–4 days, normal levels 15.7–29.6 mg/dL, severe malnutrition <8 mg/dL

   c. Serum transferrin levels: Half life 8–9 days, normal levels 200–400 mg/dL, severe malnutrition <100 mg/dL

   d. Serum retinol-binding protein: Half-life 12 hr, reflects very recent changes in protein and caloric intake. Influenced by vitamin A intake

   e. Twenty-four hours collection for urine urea nitrogen to assess nitrogen balance before and after starting nutritional therapy. Nitrogen losses are proportional to catabolic state

   f. Immunologic measurements: Absolute T-lymphocyte count, reflects visceral protein status in the absence of trauma, anesthesia, and chemotherapy, which normally depress counts. Low counts correlate with hypoalbuminemia and increased risk for sepsis

3. Anthropometric measurements

   a. Ideal body weight (IBW)

      1) Males: Height of 5 ft, ideal weight 106 lb and add 6 lb +/− 10% (frame size) for each additional inch over 5 ft

      2) Females: Height of 5 ft, ideal weight 100 lb and add 5 lb +/− 10% (frame size) for each additional inch over 5 ft

      3) Percent IBW = (actual weight/IBW) × 100, severely malnourished <69%, overweight ≥120%, morbidly obese = 200%

   b. Body mass index (BMI)

      1) Useful in diagnosis of obesity, correlated with total body fat

      2) Normal range is 19.0–26.0, patients with a BMI between 26.1 and 29.0 are considered overweight

      3) BMI >30 are considered obese

      4) Formula: BMI = Weight (Kg)/ Height (m^2)

   c. Triceps skin fold

      1) Measurements obtained using skin fold calipers on triceps of nondominant arm.

      2) Results compared with standardized tables and provide an estimate of overall subcutaneous fat stores.

4. Calculating nutritional requirements

a. Caloric requirements: Harris–Benedict equation (kcal/kg/day) calculates resting metabolic rate

   1) Men:
      66 + 13.7 (weight (kg)) + 5 (height (cm)) − 6.9 (age (yr))

   2) Women: 665 + 9.6 (weight) + 1.8 (height) − 4.7 (age)

b. Estimated caloric requirements

   1) Unstressed person: 25–35 kcal/kg/day

   2) Hospitalized patient: 35–45 kcal/kg/day

   3) Severely ill (ICU) patient: 50–70 kcal/kg/day

c. Protein requirements

   1) Maintenance: 1.0–1.5 g/kg/day

   2) Repletion: 1.5–2.0 g/kg/day

   3) Excessive loss: 2.0–2.5 g/kg/day

d. Lipid requirements

   1) Usually 25–30% of total calories

   2) Essential fatty acids are 2–4% of those calories

5. Nutritional supplements

   a. Enteral feeding is the preferred method of nutritional supplementation. Whenever possible feed the gut

      1) Enteral feeding maintains gut integrity, reduces the risk of sepsis from gut bacteria

      2) May be administered orally, per nasogastric, gastrostomy, or jejunostomy tube. All carry the risk of aspiration, but jejunostomy has the lowest risk

      3) May be continuous or intermittent bolus feedings

      4) Least expensive, most convenient

   b. Parenteral feeding

      1) Useful when patient is on bowel rest, and gut should not or can't be fed

      2) Total parenteral nutrition (TPN) requires central venous access. Solutions are a hyperosmolar mixture of dextrose, amino acids, vitamins, minerals, trace elements, electrolytes, and in some institutions fat emulsions are also directly added to mixture

      3) Provides patients with all the necessary daily requirements

4) Monitor patients carefully when starting TPN. Electrolytes, liver enzymes, white count, and fluid status. These patients are at high risk for hyperglycemia, infection, hypophosphatemia, hyponatremia, hepatic steatosis, and biliary disease

5) When discontinuing TPN you should slowly taper the person off of TPN. This will prevent hypoglycemia by allowing patients insulin levels to slowly return to normal

TABLE 19	Vitamins and Minerals	
NUTRIENT	**DEFICIENCY**	**EXCESS**
B₁ (thiamine)	Dry beriberi → neuropathy Wet beriberi → high-output cardiac failure Either → Wernicke-Korsakoff' s syndrome	
B₂ (riboflavin)		Cheilosis (mouth fissures)
B₃ (niacin)	Pellagra → dementia, diarrhea, dermatitis. Also seen in Hartnup's disease (dz of tryptophan metabolism)	
B₅ (pantothenate)		Enteritis, dermatitis
B₆ (pyridoxine)	Neuropathy (frequently caused by isoniazid therapy for TB)	
B₁₂ (Cyanocobalamin)	Pernicious anemia (lack of intrinsic factor) → neuropathy, megaloblastic anemia, glossitis	
Biotin	Dermatitis, enteritis (caused by ↑ consumption of raw eggs, due to the avidin in the raw eggs blocking biotin absorption)	
Chromium	Glucose intolerance (cofactor for insulin)	
Copper	Leukopenia, bone demineralization	
Folic acid	Neural tube defects, megaloblastic anemia	
Iodine	Hypothyroidism, cretinism, goiter	

TABLE 19	*Continued*	
NUTRIENT	**DEFICIENCY**	**EXCESS**
Iron	Plummer-Vinson syndrome = esophageal webs, Spoon Nails	Hemochromatosis → multiorgan failure (bronze diabetes)
Selenium	Myopathy (Keshan's disease, see Appendix A)	
Vitamin A	Metaplasia of respiratory epithelia (seen in cystic fibrosis due to failure of fat-soluble vitamin absorption), xerophthalmia, night blindness (lack of retinal in rod cells), acne, Bitot's spots, frequent respiratory infections (respiratory epithelial defects)	Pseudotumor cerebri (can be caused by consuming polar bear livers), headache, nausea, vomiting, skin peeling
Vitamin C	Scurvy: poor wound healing, hypertrophic bleeding gums, easy bruising, deficient osteoid mimicking rickets	
Vitamin D	Rickets in kids, osteomalacia in adults	Kidney stones, dementia, constipation, abdominal pain, depression
Vitamin E	Fragile RBCs, sensory & motor peripheral neuropathy	
Vitamin K	Clotting deficiency	
Zinc	Poor wound healing, decreased taste & smell, alopecia, diarrhea, dermatitis, depression (similar to pellagra)	
Calories	**Marasmus** = total calorie malnutrition → pts look deceptively well, but immunosuppressed, poor wound healing, impaired growth	
Protein	**Kwashiorkor** = protein malnutrition → edema/ascites, immunosuppression, poor wound healing, impaired growth & development	

XV. TOXICOLOGY

TABLE 20	Toxicology		
TOXIN	**SI/SX**	**DX**	**ANTIDOTE**
Acetaminophen	Nausea/vomiting within 2 hr, ↑ liver enzymes, ↑ prothrombin time at 24–48 hr	Blood level	N-acetylcysteine within 8–10 hr
Alkali agents	Derived from batteries, dishwasher detergent, drain cleaners, ingestion causes mucosal burns → dysphagia & drooling	Clinical	Milk or water, then NPO
Anticholinergic	**Dry as a bone, mad as a hatter, blind as a bat, hot as a hare** (delirium, miosis, fever)	Clinical	Physostigmine
Arsenic	**Mees lines** (white horizontal stripes on fingernails), capillary leak, seizures	Blood level	Gastric lavage & dimercaprol
Aspirin	Tinnitus, respiratory alkalosis, **anion gap metabolic acidosis with normal S_{OSM}**[a]	Blood level	Bicarbonate, dialysis
Benzodiazepine	Rapid onset of weakness, ataxia, drowsiness	Blood level	Flumazenil
β-Blockers	Bradycardia, heart block, obtundation, **hyperkalemia, hypoglycemia**	Clinical	Glucagon, IV calcium
Carbon monoxide	Dyspnea, confusion, coma, **cherry-red color of skin**, mucosal cyanosis	Carboxy-Hgb[b]	100% O_2 or hyperbaric O_2
Cyanide	In seconds to minutes → trismus, **almond-scented breath**, coma	Blood level	Amyl nitrite ⊕ Na thiosulfate
Digoxin	**Change in color vision, supraventricular tacyhcardia with heart block**, vomiting	Blood level[c]	Anti-digoxin Fab-antibodies
Ethylene glycol	**Calcium oxalate crystals in urine, anion gap metabolic acidosis with high S_{OSM}**[a]	Blood level	Ethanol drip, fomepizole[d]

TABLE 20	*Continued*		
TOXIN	**SI/SX**	**DX**	**ANTIDOTE**
Heparin	Bleeding, thrombocytopenia	Clinical	Protamine
Iron	Vomiting, bloody diarrhea, acidosis, CXR → radiopaque tablets	Blood level	Deferoxamine
Isoniazid	Confusion, peripheral neuropathy	Blood level	Pyridoxine
Lead	**Microcytic anemia with basophilic stippling,** ataxia, retardation, peripheral neuropathy, **purple lines on gums**	Blood level	EDTA, penicillamine
Mercury	**"Erethism"** = ↓ **memory, insomnia, timidity, delirium (mad as a hatter)**	Blood level	Ipacac, dimercaprol
Methanol	**Anion gap metabolic acidosis with high S_{OSM},**[a] **blindness, optic disk hyperemia**	Blood level	Ethanol drip, bicarbonate
Opioids	CNS/respiratory depression, miosis	Blood level	Narcan
Organophosphate	Incontinence, cough, wheezing, dyspnea, miosis, bradycardia, heart block, tremor	Blood level	Atropine, pralidoxime
Phenobarbitol	CNS depression, hypothermia, miosis, hypotensions	Blood level	Charcoal, bicarbonate
Quinidine	Torsades des pointes (ventricular tachycardia)	Blood level	IV magnesium
Theophylline	First Sx = hematemesis, then CNS → seizures or coma, cardiac → arrhythmias, hypotension	Blood level[c]	Ipecac, charcoal, cardiac monitor
Tricyclics	Anticholinergic Sx, QRS >100 ms, torsades des pointes	Blood level	Bicarbonate drip
Warfarin	Bleeding	↑ PT	Vitamin K

[a]S_{OSM} = serum osmolality.
[b]carboxyhemoglobin.
[c]correlates in acute but not chronic toxicity.
[d]see *N Engl J Med* 1999, 340:832–838.

TABLE 21	Fish and Shellfish Toxins

Ciguatera

1. Most common fish-borne illness worldwide and the most common type of nonbacterial food poisoning reported in the US
2. Species of fish include barracuda, grouper, snapper, and sea bass
3. The bigger the fish, the higher the concentration of ciguatoxin
4. Ciguatoxin has anticholinesterase and cholinergic properties, its toxicity is related to the competitive inhibition of calcium-regulated cell membrane sodium channels
5. Sxs: Begin within 6 hr of eating a Ciguatoxic fish
   a) GI complaints: vomiting, watery diarrhea, abdominal cramps, lasts 24–48 hr
   b) Neurologic symptoms: paresthesia of lips and extremities, reversal of hot-cold sensation, vertigo, blurred vision, tremor, ataxia, feeling of loose painful teeth. May persist for months and are aggravated by alcohol consumption or stress.
   c) Shock: hypotension, respiratory failure
6. Tx: prevention, supportive measures. IV Mannitol can be given for severe cases, and amitryptiline for parasthesias

Scombroid

1. A histaminelike reaction associated with marine tuna, mackerel, jacks, dolphin (mahi-mahi), and bluefish
2. Scombrotoxin formed when surface bacteria Proteus and Klebsiella on the fish secrete the enzyme histidine decarboxylase and convert histidine in the fish flesh to histamine. This and other histamine like substances act to produce the clinical effects
3. Sxs: flushing hot sensation of face and neck, pruritis, urticaria, headache, dizziness, burning sensation in mouth and throat, bronchospasm, angioedema and hypotension can occur
4. Tx: supportive, antihistamines, cimetidine, epinephrine, corticosteroids

Paralytic Shellfish

1. Caused by ingestion of mollusks (mussels, clams, oysters, and scallops) that have concentrated the *Saxitoxin*
2. Sxs: Parasthesias of mouth and extremities, sensation of floating, ataxia, vertigo, and muscle paralysis (generalized peripheral nerve dysfunction)
3. Fatality rate of 8–9%, with deaths occurring in 1–12 hr secondary to respiratory failure
4. *Saxitoxin* acts by inhibiting sodium channels in nerve terminals blocking nerve and muscle action potential propagation
5. Tx: supportive, no known antidote, protect airway, and consider mechanical ventilation

TABLE 21	*Continued*

Neurotoxic Shellfish

1. Caused by ingestion of mollusks that have concentrated the *Brevitoxin*
2. Sxs: not as bad as paralytic shellfish, parasthesis like those seen in ciguatera poisoning (hot/cold reversal), vomiting, diarrhea, no paralysis or respiratory failure. Self limited
3. Aerosolized *Brevitoxin* during a red tide at the beach can cause rhinorrhea, conjunctivitis, bronchospasm, and cough
4. *Brevitoxin* acts on the sodium channels of postganglionic cholinergic nerve fibers to inhibit transmission in skeletal muscle
5. Tx: supportive and symptomatic

Tetrodotoxin

1. Rare in United States. Caused by eating Japanese puffer fish (*Fugu*), blue ringed octopus, newts, and salamanders
2. Sxs: begin within minutes of ingestion, parasthesias of face and extremities, salivation, hyperemesis, weakness, ataxia, dysphagia, ascending paralysis, respiratory failure, hypotension, bradycardia, fixed dilated pupils
3. Tetrodotoxinis chemically related to saxitoxin causing a similar blockade of sodium channels in nerve terminals. There are also direct effects of the toxin on the medulla, and reversible competitive blockade at the motor end plate
4. Tx: Supportive, airway and ventilatory support, anticholinesterase inhibitors, i.e., edrophonium. Prognosis is good if patient survives first 24 hr

Source: **Arch Intern Med, Vol 149, Aug 1989, 1735–1740**

TABLE 22	Bites and Stings	
BITE OR STING	**SYMPTOMS**	**TREATMENT**
Bee/Wasp	Local Inflammation or Anaphylactic Reaction possible	Scrape out stinger if present. Wash with soap and water. **Airway**, IV fluids, O$_2$, Cardiac monitoring for systemic effects. **Epinephrine** (1:1000) 0.3–0.5 ml SQ in adults, 0.01 ml/kg in peds May be given a second time in 10–15 min. **Diphenhydramine** 25–50 mg IV/IM. **Methylprednisilone**: 80–120 mg IV. Prednisone taper upon stabilization
Black Widow ("red hourglass" on abdomen)	Sharp pain at site. Deep burning, aching pain along extremity. Vomiting, headache, chest tightness, and hypertension. Rigid Abdominal muscles	**Airway**, IV fluids, O$_2$, Cardiac monitoring for systemic effects. Antivenin can be given, skin test prior to administration. Nitrates for hypertension. Wound care, Tetanus prophylaxis, Pain relief

TABLE 22	*Continued*	
BITE OR STING	**SYMPTOMS**	**TREATMENT**
Brown Recluse Spider ("brown-yellow violin" on thorax)	Pain at site, nausea, myalgias and arthralgias Fever, chills, rash, necrosis at bite site	Wound care and ice congresses Erythromycin P.O. Plastic surgery consult for significant necrosis
Snake (depends on geographical region)	Fang puncture marks, vomiting, diarrhea, restlessness, dysphagia, muscle weakness, fasciculations, generalized bleeding	ACLS resuscitation as needed. Type specific antivenin. Tetanus prophylaxis, monitor for compartment syndrome of affected extremity
Cats	Tender regional lymphadenopathy. Local edema, erythema, decreased range of motion (tenosynovitis). *Pasteurella* commonly involved	Copious irrigation and wound care. Augmentin P.O., IV Antibiotics for immunocompromised. Tetanus prophylaxis. Close follow up
Dogs	Local edema and erythema. *Pasteurella* also commonly involved, assess nature of bite, unprovoked worrisome for Rabies, provoked → unlikely Rabies	Copious irrigation and wound care. Tetanus prophylaxis. Rule out fractures. Augmentin P.O.
Human	Treat all knuckle injuries in a fight as a human bite. Erythema, edema, purulence, pain, fever, and chills. Aerobic and anaerobic bacteria commonly involved	Copious irrigation, Tetanus prophylaxis, Augmentin P.O., IV antibiotics for severe unresolving infection or in immunocompromised. Rule out fractures. Close follow up

XVI. COMMON OUTPATIENT COMPLAINTS AND TREATMENTS

A. Headache

1. **Signs/symptoms & differential diagnosis (Table 23)**

TABLE 23	Summary of Headaches	

TYPE	EPIDEMIO-LOGY	CHARACTERISTICS
Tension	Usually after age 20 (rarely >age 50)	• Most common headache type • **Bilateral, bandlike, dull in quality** • Worse with stress; not aggravated by activity • Chronic HA associated with depression
Cluster	Male:female = 6:1 Mean age 30 yr	• **Unilateral,** stabbing peri/retro-orbital pain, lasting 15 min to 3 hr • Seasonal attacks occur in series (6x/day) lasting weeks, followed by months of remission • **Associated with ipsilateral lacrimation (85%), ptosis, nasal congestion & rhinorrhea** • Often occurs within 90 min of onset of sleep
Migraine	80% have positive FHx **Female:male =** 3:1	• Classically, HA is **unilateral (60%)** with **aura (only 15%);** pt looks for quiet place to rest • Visual aura: **scotoma** (blind spots), **teichopsia** (jagged zigzag lines), **photopsias** (shimmering lights), or **rhodopsins** (colors) • Accompanied by **nausea & photophobia** • Triggered by stress, odors, certain foods, alcohol, menstruation, or sleep deprivation
Temporal arteritis (Giant cell)	Female:male = 2:1 Age >50	• **Unilateral temporal** headache • **Associated with jaw claudication, temporal artery tenderness with palpation, ESR ≥50** • 50% also have polymyalgia rheumatica • If not treated leads to optic neuritis & **blindness** • Screen by ESR; Dx with temporal artery Bx
Trigeminal neuralgia	Peak age at 60	• Episodic, severe pain shooting from side of mouth to ipsilateral ear, eye, or nose
Withdrawal headache		• Common cause of frequent headaches • Can be withdrawal from various drugs
SAH*		• Head trauma is most common cause • Spontaneous: usually berry aneurysm rupture • Classically the "worst headache of my life"

*Subarachnoid hemorrhage.

2. **Dx is made by clinical history & physical, except:**

   a. **Temporal arteritis Dx requires temporal artery biopsy**

   b. **Trigeminal neuralgia Dx requires head CT or MRI** to rule

TABLE 24	Treatment of Headaches
HEADACHE	**TREATMENT**
Tension	• Acutely NSAIDs or Midrin® • Prophylaxis with antidepressants or β-blockers
Cluster	• Acutely 100% O_2, sumatriptan∗ or dihydroergotamine • Prophylaxis with verapamil, lithium, methysergide, or ergotamine
Migraine	• Acutely sumatriptan,∗ dihydroergotamine, NSAIDs, antiemetics • Prophylaxis with β-blockers (first line) or calcium blockers
Temporal arteritis	• High-dose prednisone or cytotoxic drug to prevent blindness
Trigeminal neuralgia	• Carbamazepine (first line), phenytoin, clonazepam, valproate
Withdrawal	• NSAIDs
SAH	• Immediate neurosurgical evaluation & nimodipine to reduce incidence of postrupture vasospasm & ischemia

∗Sumatriptan contraindicated with known coronary dz or ergot drugs taken within 24 hr.

out sinusitis, cerebellopontine angle neoplasm, multiple sclerosis, herpes zoster

c. **Subarachnoid hemorrhage requires** confirmation by CT scan or lumbar puncture to detect CSF xanthochromia (can be detected 6 hr after onset of HA)

d. Suspect intracranial lesion causing headache in **pts > 50 or pts with headaches immediately upon waking up**

e. **Suspect ↑ ICP in pts awakened in middle of night by headache, who have projectile vomiting, or focal neural deficits; obtain head CT**

3. **Treatment (Table 24)**

B. Ears, Nose, and Throat

1. Otitis externa

a. Si/Sx = **pulling on pinna or pushing on tragus causes pain**

b. *Pseudomonas* causes malignant otitis externa in diabetics

c. Tx = antibiotic ear drops

d. DDx = Ramsay Hunt syndrome (herpes zoster oticus)

1) Herpes infection of geniculate ganglia (CN VII)

2) Si/Sx = painful vesicles in external auditory meatus

3) Tx = urgent acyclovir to prevent extension to meningitis

  e. In diabetics, get CT/MRI of temporal bone to rule out **malignant otitis externa**, which requires surgical débridement

2. Epistaxis

  a. Ninety percent of bleeds occur at Kiesselbach's plexus (anterior nasal septum)

  b. **No. 1 cause of epistaxis in children is trauma (induced by exploring digits)**

  c. Also precipitated by rhinitis, nasal mucosa dryness, septal deviation & bone spurs, alcohol, antiplatelet medication, bleeding diathesis

  d. Tx = direct pressure, topical nasal vasoconstrictors (Neosynephrine), consider anterior nasal packing if unable to stop, 5% originate in posterior nasal cavity requiring packing to occlude choanae

3. Sinusitis (Table 25)

  a. Maxillary sinuses most commonly involved

  b. Dx = CT scan showing inflammatory changes or bone destruction

TABLE 25	Sinusitis		
	ORGANISMS	**Si/Sx**	**Tx**
Acute bacterial (<4 wk)	*S. pneumoniae, H. influenzae, Moraxella catarrhalis*	**Purulent rhinorrhea,** headache, **pain on sinus palpation,** fever, **halitosis,** anosmia, **tooth pain**	Bactrim or amoxicillin, decongestants
Chronic bacterial (>3 mo)	*Bacteroides, Staph. aureus, Pseudomonas, Streptococcus spp.*	Same as for acute but lasts longer, also otitis media in children	Surgical correction of obstruction, nasal steroids
Fungal	*Aspergillus*— **diabetics get** mucormycosis!	Usually seen in the immunocompromised	Surgery & amphotericin

TABLE 26	Pharyngitis		
DISEASE	**Si/Sx**	**Dx**	**Tx**
Group A Strep throat	High fever, **severe throat pain without cough**, edematous **tonsils with white or yellow exudate, cervical adenopathy**	• H&P 50% accurate • Antigen agglutination kit for screening • Throat swab culture is gold standard	Penicillin to prevent acute rheumatic fever
Membranous (diphtheria)	High fever, dysphagia, drooling, **can cause respiratory failure** (airway occlusion)	**Pathognomonic gray membrane on tonsils extending into throat**	**STAT antitoxin**
Fungal (*Candida*)	Dysphagia, sore throat with white, cheesy patches in oropharynx (oral thrush), **seen in AIDS & small children**	Clinical or endoscopy	Nystatin liquid, swish & swallow or fluconazole
Adenovirus	**Pharyngoconjunctival fever (fever, red eye, sore throat)**	Clinical	Supportive
Mononucleosis (EBV)	Generalized lymphadenopathy, exudative tonsillitis, palatal Petechiae & splenomegaly	• ⊕ **Heterophile antibody** • **Skin rash** occurs in pts given ampicillin	Supportive
Herpangina (coxsackie A)	Fever, pharyngitis, body ache, tender vesicles along tonsils, uvula & soft palate	Clinical	Supportive

    c. Potential complications of sinusitis include meningitis, abscess formation, orbital infection, osteomyelitis

   4. Pharyngitis (Table 26)

c. Outpatient Gastrointestinal Complaints

   1. **Dyspepsia**

     a. Si/Sx = upper abdominal pain, early satiety, postprandial abdominal bloating or distention, nausea, vomiting, often exacerbated by eating

b. DDx = peptic ulcer, gastroesophageal reflux disease (GERD), cancer, gastroparesis, malabsorption, intestinal parasite, drugs (e.g., NSAIDs), etc.

c. Dx = clinical

d. Tx = empiric for 4 wk, if Sx not relieved → endoscopy

1) Avoid caffeine, alcohol, cigarettes, NSAIDs, eat frequent small meals, stress reduction, maintain ideal body weight, elevate head of bed

2) H_2 blockers & antacids, or proton pump inhibitor

3) Antibiotics for *H. pylori* are NOT indicated for nonulcer dyspepsia

2. Gastroesophageal Reflux Disease (GERD)

a. Causes = obesity, relaxed lower esophageal sphincter, esophageal dysmotility, hiatal hernia

b. Si/Sx = heartburn occurring 30–60 min postprandial & upon reclining, usually relieved by antacid self-administration, dyspepsia, also regurgitation of gastric contents into the mouth

c. Atypical Si/Sx sometimes seen = asthma, chronic cough/laryngitis, atypical chest pain

d. Upper endoscopy → tissue damage but may be normal in 50% of cases

e. Dx = clinical, can confirm with ambulatory pH monitoring

f. Tx

1) First line = lifestyle modifications: avoid lying down postprandial, avoid spicy foods & foods that delay gastric emptying, reduction of meal size, weight loss

2) Second line = H2-receptor antagonists—aim to discontinue in 8–12 wk

3) Promotility agents may be comparable to H2-antagonists

4) Third line = proton pump inhibitors, reserve for refractory dz, often will require maintenance Tx since Sx return upon discontinuation

      5) Fourth line = surgical fundoplication, relieves Sx in 90% of pts, may be more cost-effective in younger pts or those with severe dz

  g. Sequelae

    1) Barrett's esophagus

      a) Chronic GERD → metaplasia from squamous to columnar epithelia in lower esophagus

      b) Requires close surveillance with endoscopy & aggressive Tx as 10% progress to adenocarcinoma

    2) Peptic stricture

      a) Results in gradual solid food dysphagia often with concurrent improvement of heartburn symptoms

      b) Endoscopy establishes diagnosis

      c) Requires aggressive proton pump inhibitor Tx & surgical opening if unresponsive

3. Diarrhea

  a. Diarrhea ≡ stool weight >300 g/day (normal = 100–300 g/day)

  b. Small bowel dz → stools typically voluminous, watery, & fatty

  c. Large bowel dz → stools smaller in volume but more frequent

  d. Prominent vomiting suggests viral enteritis or *Staph. aureus* food poisoning

  e. Malabsorption diarrhea characterized by high fat content

    1) Lose fat soluble vitamins, iron, calcium, & B vitamins

    2) Can cause iron deficiency, megaloblastic anemia (B_{12} loss) & hypocalcemia

  f. General Tx = oral rehydration, IV fluids, & electrolytes (supportive)

  g. Specific diarrheas (Table 27)

TABLE 27	Diarrhea		
TYPE	**CHARACTERISTICS**	**DX**	**TX**
Infectious	• **No.1 cause of acute diarrhea** • Si/Sx = vomiting, pain; blood/mucus & fevers/chills suggest invasive dz	• Stool leukocytes, Gram's stain & culture, O & P for parasitic • *C. difficile* toxin test	• Ciprofloxacin • Metronidazole for *C. difficile*[a]
Osmotic	• Causes = lactose intolerance, oral Mg, sorbitol/mannitol	• ↑ osmotic gap • Check fecal fat	• Withdraw inciting agent
Secretory	• Causes = toxins (cholera), enteric viruses, ↑ dietary fat	• Normal osmotic gap • Fasting →no change	• Supportive
Exudative	• Mucosal inflammation → plasma & serum leakage • Causes = enteritis, TB, colon CA, inflammatory bowel dz	• ↑ ESR & CRP[b] • Radiologic imaging or colonoscopy to visualize intestine	• Varies by cause —see appropriate section of text
Rapid transit	• Causes = laxatives, surgical excision of intestinal tissue	• Hx of surgery or laxative use	• Supportive
Encopresis	• Oozing around fecal impaction in children or sick elderly	• History of constipation	• Fiber rich diet & laxatives
Celiac sprue	• Gluten allergy (wheat, barley, rye, oats contain gluten) • Sx/Si = weakness, failure to thrive, growth retardation • Classic rash = **dermatitis herpetiformis** = pruritic, red papulovesicular lesions on shoulders, elbows & knees • 10–15% of pts develop intestinal lymphoma	**Dx by small bowel biopsy → pathognomonic blunting of intestinal villi**	• Avoid dietary gluten

TABLE 27	*Continued*		
TYPE	**CHARACTERISTICS**	**DX**	**TX**
Tropical sprue	• Diarrhea probably caused by a tropical infection • Si/Sx = glossitis, diarrhea, weight loss, steatorrhea	Dx = clinical	Tetracycline ⊕ folate
Whipple's disease	• GI infection by *Tropheryma whippelii* • Si/Sx = diarrhea, arthritis, rash, anemia	Dx = biopsy → PAS⊕ macrophages in intestines	Penicillin or tetracycline
Lactase deficiency	• Most of world is lactase deficient as adults, people lose as they emerge from adolescence Si/Sx = abdominal pain, • diarrhea, flatulence after ingestion of any lactose-containing product	Dx = clinical	Avoid lactose or take exogenous lactase
Intestinal lymphangiec-tasia	• Seen in children, congenital or acquired dilation of intestinal lymphatics leads to marked GI protein loss • Si/Sx = diarrhea, hypoproteinemia, edema	Dx = jejunal biopsy	Supportive
Pancreas dz	• Typically seen in pancreatitis & cystic fibrosis due to deficiency of pancreatic digestive enzymes • Si/Sx = foul smelling steatorrhea, megaloblastic anemia (folate deficiency), weight loss	Hx of prior pancreatic disease	Pancrease supplementa-tion

[a]Vancomycin reserved for resistance.
[b]CRP = C-reactive protein.

    h. Common infectious pathogens for diarrhea (Table 28)

D. **Urogenital Complaints**

    1. Urinary Tract Infection (UTI)

        a. Epidemiology

            1) Forty percent of females have ≥1UTI, 8% have bacteri-uria at a given time

TABLE 28	Infectious Causes of Diarrhea		
	BACTERIAL	**VIRAL**	**PARASITIC**
Etiology	*E. coli, Shigella, Salmonella, Campylobacter jejuni, Vibrio parahaemolyticus, Vibrio cholera, Yersinia enterocolitica*	Rotavirus Norwalk virus	*Giardia lamblia, Cryptosporidium, Entamoeba histolytica*
Tx	Ciprofloxacin, Bactrim	Supportive	Metronidazole

2) Most common in sexually active young women, elderly, posturethral catheter or instrumentation—rare in males ($\uparrow$ risk with prostate dz)

3) Due to *E. coli* (80%), *S. saprophyticus* (15%), other gram-negative rods

b. Si/Sx = **burning during urination**, urgency, sense of incomplete bladder emptying, hematuria, lower abdominal pain, nocturia

c. Systemic Sx = fever, chills, **back pain suggest pyelonephritis**

d. Dx = **UA** → **pyuria**; $\oplus$ bacteria on Gram's stain; positive culture results

e. Tx

1) Lower UTI → Bactrim (first line), fluoroquinolone for refractory dz

2) Uncomplicated pyelonephritis → same antibiotics given IV or PO depending on severity of pt's illness

3) Men cured within 7 days of Tx do not warrant further work-up, but **adolescents & men with pyelonephritis or recurrent infxn require renal Utz & intravenous pyelogram to rule out anatomic etiology**

4) UTI 2° to bacterial prostatitis requires 6–12 wk of antibiotics

5) Asymptomatic bacteriuria

a) Defined as urine culture >100,000 CFU/mL but no Sx

b) Only Tx in 1) pregnancy (use penicillins or nitrofurantoin), or pts with 2) renal transplant, 3) about to undergo GU procedure, 4) severe vesicular-ureteral reflux, & 5) struvite calculi

2. Sexually Transmitted Diseases (STDs)—See Section C for AIDS (Table 29)

TABLE 29	Sexually Transmitted Diseases	
DISEASE	**CHARACTERISTICS**	**Tx**
Herpes simplex virus (HSV)	• Most common cause of genital ulcers (causes 60–70% of cases) • Si/Sx = **painful vesicular & ulcerated** lesions 1–3 mm diameter, onsets 3–7 days after exposure • Lesions generally resolve over 7 days • Primary infection also characterized by malaise, low grade fever & inguinal adenopathy in 40% of patients • Recurrent lesions are similar appearing, but milder in severity & shorter in duration, lasting about 2–5 days • Dx confirmed with direct fluorescent antigen (DFA) staining, Tzanck prep, serology, HSV PCR, or culture	• Tx = acyclovir, famciclovir, or valacyclovir to ↓ duration of viral shedding & shorten initial course
Pelvic inflammatory disease	• *Chlamydia trachomatis* & *Neisseria gonorrhoeae* are primary pathogens, but PID is polymicrobial involving both aerobic & anaerobic bacteria • PID includes endometritis, salpingitis, tuboovarian abscess (TOA) & pelvic peritonitis • Infertility occurs in 15% of pts after one episode of salpingitis, ↑ to 75% after ≥three episodes • Risk of ectopic pregnancy ↑ 7–10 times in women with history of salpingitis • Dx = abdominal, adnexal & cervical motion tenderness + at least one of the following: ⊕ Gram's stain, temp >38° C, WBC >10,000, pus on culdocentesis or laparoscopy, tuboovarian abscess on bimanual or Utz	• Toxic pts, ↓ immunity & noncompliant should be Tx as inpatients with IV antibiotics • Use fluoroquinolone + metronidazole or cephalosporin + doxycycline • Start antibiotic as soon as PID is suspected, even before culture results are available

TABLE 29	*Continued*	
DISEASE	**CHARACTERISTICS**	**Tx**
Human papilloma-virus (HPV)	• Serotypes 16, 18 most commonly associated with cervical cancer • Incubation period varies from 6 wk to 3 mo, spread by direct skin-to-skin contact • Infection after single contact with an infected individual results in 65% transmission rate • Si/Sx = condyloma acuminata (genital warts) = soft, fleshy growths on vulva, vagina, cervix, perineum & anus • Dx = clinical, confirmed with biopsy	• Topical podophyllin or trichloracetic acid, if refractory → cryosurgery or excision • If pregnant, C-section recommended to avoid vaginal lacerations
Syphilis (*Treponema pallidum*)	• Si/Sx = **painless ulcer** with bilateral inguinal adenopathy, chancre heals in 3–9 wk • Because of lack of Sx, Dx of primary syphilis is often missed • 4–8 wk after appearance of chancre, 2° dz → fever, lymphadenopathy, maculopapular rash affecting palms & soles, condyloma lata in intertriginous areas • Dx = serologies, VDRL & RPR for screening, FTA-ABS to confirm	• Benzathine penicillin G

3. Acquired Immunodeficiency Syndrome (AIDS)

   a. Epidemiology

      1) AIDS is a global pandemic (currently the fastest spread is in SE Asia & central Europe)

      2) **Heterosexual transmission is the most common mode worldwide**

      3) In the US, IV drug users & their sex partners are the fastest growing population of HIV⊕ patients

      4) Homosexual transmission is slowing dramatically [see *N Engl J Med* 1999, 341:1046–1050]

   b. HIV biology

      1) Retrovirus with the usual *gag, pol,* & *env* genes

2) p24 is a core protein encoded by *gag* gene, can be used clinically to follow disease progression

3) gp120 & gp41 are envelope glycoproteins that are produced on cleavage of gp160, coded by *env*

4) Reverse transcriptase (coded by *pol*) converts viral RNA to DNA so it can integrate into the host's DNA

5) Cellular entry is by binding to both CD4 & an additional ligand (can be CCR4, CCR5, others) that typically is a cytokine receptor

6) HIV can infect CD4⊕ T cells, macrophages, thymic cells, astrocytes, dendritic cells, & others

7) The mechanisms of T-cell destruction are not well understood but probably include direct cell lysis, induction of CTL responses against infected CD4⊕ cells, & exhaustion of bone marrow production (suppression of production of T cells)

8) In addition, the virus induces alterations in host cytokine patterns rendering surviving lymphocytes ineffective

c. Disease course

1) In most patients, AIDS is relentlessly progressive, & death occurs within 10–15 yr of HIV infection

2) Long-term survivors

a) Up to 5% of patients are "long-term survivors," meaning the disease does not progress even after 15–20 yr without Tx

b) This may be due to infection with defective virus, a potent host immune response, or genetic resistance of the host

c) People with homozygous deletions of CCR5 or other viral coreceptors are highly resistant to infection with HIV, while heterozygotes are less resistant

3) Although patients can have no clinical evidence of disease for many years, **HIV has no latent phase in its life cycle**; clinical silence in those patients who eventually progress is due to daily, temporarily successful host repopulation of T cells

4) Death is usually caused by opportunistic infections (OIs)

a) OIs typically onset after CD4 counts fall below 200

b) Below 200 CD4 cells, all pts should be on permanent

Bactrim prophylaxis against *P. carinii* pneumonia (PCP) & *Toxoplasma encephalitis*

c) Below 75 CD4 cells, all patients should receive azithromycin prophylaxis against *M. avium-intracellulare* complex (MAC)

d) Kaposi's sarcoma = common skin cancer found in homosexual HIV patients, thought to be caused by cotransmission of human herpes virus 8 (HHV 8)

e) Other diseases found in AIDS patients include generalized wasting & dementia

d. Treatment

1) Triple combination therapy is now the cornerstone

a) Cocktail includes two nucleoside analogues (e.g., AZT, ddI, d4T) ⊕ a protease inhibitor

b) Protease inhibitors block the splicing of the large *gag* precursor protein into its final components, p24 & p7

c) Newest addition to arsenal is hydroxyurea

i) Inhibits host ribonucleotide reductase → decreased concentration of purines

ii) ddI is a purine analogue (competitor), so hydroxyurea ↑ efficacy of ddI

iii) In theory, virus should not be able to become resistant to hydroxyurea, since it acts on a host enzyme, & not on the virus

2) **No patient should ever be on any single drug regimen for HIV—resistance is invariable in monotherapy**

3) Current Tx is able to suppress viral replication to below detectable limits in the majority of patients, but **up to 50% of patients end up "failing" therapy (viral loads rebound)**

4) **Failure of the regimen is associated with poor compliance** (missed doses lead to resistance) & **prior exposure to one or more drugs in the regimen** (the virus is already resistant to the agent)

5) The long-term significance of viral suppression is unclear, but **it is known that the virus is NOT cleared from the body at up to 2 yr after it ceases to be detectable in the blood** (it can be found latent in lymph nodes)

4. Hematuria

    a. Red/brown urine discoloration 2° to RBCs, correlates with presence of >5 RBCs/high-powered field on microanalysis

    b. Can be painful or painless

        1) Painless = 1° renal dz (tumor, glomerulonephritis), TB infection, vesicular dz (bladder tumor), prostatic dz

        2) Painful = nephrolithiasis, renal infarction, UTI

    c. DDx = myoglobinuria or hemoglobinuria, where hemoglobin dipstick is positive but no RBCs are seen on microanalysis

    d. Dx = finding of RBCs in urinary sediment

        1) Urinalysis → WBCs (infection) or RBC casts (glomerulonephritis)

        2) CBC → anemia (renal failure), polycythemia (renal cell CA)

        3) Urogram will show nephrolithiasis & tumors (Utz → cystic vs. solid)

        4) Cystoscopy only after UA & IVP; best for lower urinary tract

    e. Tx varies by cause

5. Prostate

    a. Benign prostatic hyperplasia

        1) Hyperplasia of the periurethral prostrate causing bladder outlet obstruction

        2) Common after age 45 (autopsy shows that 90% of men over 70 have BPH)

        3) Does not predispose to prostrate cancer

        4) Si/Sx urinary frequency, urgency, nocturia, ↓ size & force of urinary stream leading to hesitancy & intermittency, sensation of incomplete emptying, worsening to continuous overflow incontinence or urinary retention, rectal exam → enlarged prostate (classically a rubbery vs. firm, hard gland that may suggest prostate cancer) with loss of median furrow

        5) Labs → PSA elevated in up to 50% of pts, not specific—not useful marker for BPH

        6) Dx based on symptomatic scoring system, i.e., prostate size >30 mL (determined by Utz or exam), maximum

urinary flow rate (<10 mL/sec) & postvoid residual urine volume (>50 mL) (see *J Urology* 1992, 148:1549)

7) Tx = a-blocker (e.g., terazosin), 5-a-reductase inhibitor (e.g., Finasteride); avoid anticholinergics, antihistaminergics, or narcotics

8) Refractory dz requires surgery = transurethral resection of prostate (TURP); open prostatectomy recommended for larger glands (>75 g)

b. Prostatitis

1) Si/Sx = fever, chills, low back pain, urinary frequency & urgency, tender, possible fluctuant & swollen prostate

2) Labs → leukocytosis, pyuria, bacteriuria

3) Dx = clinical

4) Tx = systemic antibiotics

6. Impotence

a. Affects 30 million men in the US, strongly associated with age (about 40% among 40-yr-olds & 70% among 70-yr-olds)

b. Causes

1) 1° erectile dysfunction = never been able to sustain erections

a) Psychological (sexual guilt, fear of intimacy, depression, anxiety)

b) ↓ testosterone 2° to hypothalamic-pituitary-gonadal disorder

c) Hypo- or hyperthyroidism, Cushing's syndrome, ↑ prolactin

2) 2° erectile dysfunction = acquired, >**90% due to organic cause**

a) Vascular dz = atherosclerosis of penile arteries and/or venous leaks causing inadequate impedance of venous outflow

b) Drugs = diuretics, clonidine, CNS depressants, tricyclic antidepressants, high-dose anticholinergics, antipsychotics

c) Neurologic dz = stroke, temporal lobe seizures, multiple sclerosis, spinal cord injury, autonomic dysfunction 2° to diabetes, post-TURP or open prostatic surgery

c. Dx

    1) Clinical, rule out above organic causes

    2) **Nocturnal penile tumescence** testing differentiates psychogenic from organic—nocturnal tumescence is involuntary, ⊕ in psychogenic but not in organic dz

d. Tx

    1) Sildenafil (Viagra)

        a) Selective inhibitor of cGMP specific phosphodiesterase type 5a → improves relaxation of smooth muscles in corpora cavernosa

        b) Side effects = transient headache, flushing, dyspepsia & rhinitis, transient visual disturbances (blue hue) is very rare, drug may lower blood pressure → **use of nitrates is an absolute contraindication,** deaths have resulted from combo

    2) Vacuum-constriction devices use negative pressure to draw blood into penis with band placed at base of penis to retain erection

    3) Intracavernosal prostaglandin injection has mean duration about 60 min; risks = penile bruising/bleeding & priapism

    4) Surgery = penile prostheses implantation; venous or arterial surgery

    5) Testosterone therapy for hypogonadism

    6) Behavioral therapy, & counseling for depression & anxiety

E. Gynecology

1. Menstrual cycle

  a. Due to hypothalamic pulses of gonadotropin releasing hormone (GnRH), pituitary release of follicle stimulating hormone (FSH) & luteinizing hormone (LH), & ovarian sex steroids estradiol & progesterone

  b. ↑ or ↓ of any of these hormones → irregular menses or amenorrhea

  c. At birth, the human ovary contains approximately 1 million primordial follicles each with an oocyte arrested in the prophase stage of meiosis

  d. Process of ovulation begins in puberty = follicular maturation

    1) After ovulation, the dominant follicle released becomes

the corpus luteum, which secretes progesterone to prepare the endometrium for possible implantation

2) If the ovum is not fertilized, the corpus luteum undergoes involution, menstruation begins, & cycle repeats

2. Contraception

a. Oral contraceptive pills (OCPs) = combination estrogen & progestin

1) Progestin is major contraceptive by suppressing LH & thus ovulation, also thickens cervical mucus so it is less favorable to semen

2) Estrogen participates by suppressing FSH thereby preventing selection & maturation of a dominant follicle

3) Estrogen & progesterone together inhibit implantation by thinning endometrial lining, also resulting in light or missed menses

4) Monophasic pills deliver a constant dose of estrogen & progestin

5) Phasic OCPs alter this ratio (usually by varying the dose of progestin) that slightly ↓ the total dose of hormone per month, but also has slightly ↑ rate of breakthrough bleeding between periods

6) Pts usually resume fertility once OCPs are discontinued; however, 3% may have prolonged postpill amenorrhea

7) Absolute contraindications to use of OCPs = pregnancy, DVT or thromboembolic dz, endometrial CA, cerebrovascular or coronary artery dz, breast CA, cigarette smoking in women >35 yr old, hepatic dz/neoplasm, abnormal vaginal bleeding, hyperlipidemia

3. Pap smear

a. First Pap smear should be done when woman becomes sexually active or by age 18, then yearly thereafter

b. In pts with one sexual partner, three consecutive normal Pap smears, & onset of sexual activity after age 25, may be able to screen less frequently

c. Reliability depends on presence/absence of cervical inflammation, adequacy of specimen, & prompt fixation of specimen to avoid artifact

d. If Pap → mild- or low-grade atypia → repeat Pap, atypia may spontaneously regress

    e. Recurrent mild atypia or high-grade atypia → more intensive evaluation

1. Colposcopy

    a) Allows for magnification of cervix, permitting subtle areas of dysplastic change to be visualized, optimizing selection of biopsy sites

    b) Cervix washed with acetic acid solution, white areas, abnormally vascularized areas, & punctate lesions are selected for biopsy

2. Endocervical curettage (ECC) → sample of endocervix obtained at same time of colposcopy so that disease further up endocervical canal may be detected

3. Cone biopsy

    a) Cone-shaped specimen encompassing squamocolumnar junction (SCJ) & any lesions on ectocervix removed from cervix by knife, laser, or wire loop

    b) Allows for more complete ascertainment of extent of disease, and in many cases, is therapeutic as well as diagnostic

    c) Indications = ≈ ECC, unsatisfactory colposcopy meaning that entire scquamocolumnar junction was not visualized, & discrepancy between Pap smear & colposcopy biopsy

    f. Tx = excision of premalignant or malignant lesions—if cancer, see Section VIII below for appropriate adjunctive modalities

4. Vaginitis

    a. Fifty percent of cases due to *Gardnerella* ("bacterial vaginosis"), 25% due to *Trichomonas*, 25% due to *Candida* (↑ frequency in diabetics, in pregnancy & in HIV)

    b. Most common presenting symptom in vaginitis is discharge

    c. Rule out noninfectious causes, including chemical or allergic sources

    d. Dx by pelvic examination with microscopic examination of discharge

    e. DDx of vaginitis (Table 30)

5. Endometriosis

    a. Affects 1–2% of women (up to 50% in infertile women), peak age = 20–30 yr

TABLE 30	Differential Diagnosis of Vaginitis		
	CANDIDA	**TRICHOMONAS**	**GARDNERELLA**
Vaginal pH Odor Discharge	4–5 None Cheesy white	>6 Rancid Green, frothy	>5 "Fishy" on KOH prep Variable
Si/Sx	Itchy, burning erythema	Severe itching	Variable to none
Microscopy	Pseudohyphae, more pronounced on 10% KOH prep	Motile organisms	Clue cells (large epithelial cells covered with dozens of small dots)
Treatment	Fluconazole	Metronidazole— treat partner also	Metronidazole

b. Endometrial tissue in extrauterine locations, most commonly ovaries (60%), but can be anywhere in the peritoneum & rarely extraperitoneal

c. Adenomyosis = endometrial implants within the uterine wall

d. Endometrioma = endometriosis involving an ovary with implants large enough to be considered a tumor, filled with chocolate-appearing fluid (old blood) that gives them their name of "chocolate cysts"

e. Si/Sx = **the 3 D's = dysmenorrhea, dyspareunia, dyschezia** (painful defecation), pelvic pain, infertility, uterosacral nodularity palpable on rectovaginal exam, severity of Sx often do not correlate with extent of dz

f. Dx requires direct visualization via laparoscopy or laparotomy with histologic confirmation

g. Tx

1) Start with NSAIDs, can add combined estrogen & progestin pills, allowing maintenance without withdrawal bleeding & dysmenorrhea

2) Can use progestin-only pills, drawback is breakthrough bleeding

3) GnRH agonists inhibit ovarian function → hypoestrogen state

4) Danazol inhibits LH & FSH midcycle surges, side effects include hypoestrogenic & androgenic (hirsutism, acne) states

5) Conservative surgery involves excision, cauterization, or ablation of endometrial implants with preservation of ovaries & uterus

6. Recurrence after cessation of medical Tx is common, definitive Tx requires hysterectomy, ⊕ oophorectomy (TAH/BSO), lysis of adhesions, & removal of endometrial implants

7. Pts can take estrogen replacement therapy following definitive surgery, risk of reactivation of endometriosis is very small compared to risk of prolonged estrogen deficiency

F. Reproductive Endocrinology and Infertility

1. Amenorrhea

    a. Amenorrhea ≡ absence of menstruation, primary amenorrhea = a woman who has never menstruated, secondary amenorrhea = a menstrual-aged woman who has not menstruated in 6 mo

    b. Causes of amenorrhea

        1) **Pregnancy** = **most common cause**, thus every evaluation should begin with an exclusion of pregnancy before any further work-up

        2) Asherman's syndrome

            a) Scarring of the uterine cavity after a D&C procedure

            b) **The most common anatomic cause of 2° amenorrhea**

        3) Hypothalamic deficiency due to weight loss, excessive exercise (e.g., marathon runner), obesity, drug induced (e.g., marijuana, tranquilizers), malignancy (prolactinoma, craniopharyngioma), psychogenic (chronic anxiety, anorexia)

        4) Pituitary dysfunction results from either ↓ hypothalamic pulsatile release of GnRH or ↓ pituitary release of FSH or LH

        5) Ovarian dysfunction

            a) Ovarian follicles are either exhausted or resistant to stimulation by FSH & LH

            b) Si/Sx = those of estrogen deficiency = hot flashes, mood swings, vaginal dryness, dyspareunia, sleep disturbances, skin thinning

c) Note that estrogen deficiency 2° to hypothalamic-pituitary failure does not cause hot flashes, while ovarian failure does

d) Causes = inherited (e.g., Turner's syndrome), premature natural menopause, autoimmune ovarian failure (Blizzard's syndrome), alkylating chemotherapies

6) Genital outflow tract alteration, usually the result of congenital abnormalities (e.g., imperforate hymen or agenesis of uterus/vagina)

c. Tx

1) Hypothalamic → reversal of underlying cause & induction of ovulation with gonadotropins

2) Tumors → excision or bromocriptine for prolactinoma

3) Genital tract obstruction → surgery if possible

4) Ovarian dysfunction → exogenous estrogen replacement

2. Dysfunctional uterine bleeding

a. Irregular menstruation without anatomic lesions of the uterus

b. **Usually due to chronic estrogen stimulation** (vs. amenorrhea, an estrogen deficient state), more rarely to genital outflow tract obstruction

c. Abnormal bleeding = bleeding at intervals <21 days or >36 days, lasting longer than 7 days, or blood loss >80 mL

d. Menorrhagia (excessive bleeding) is usually due to anovulation

e. Dx

1) Rule out anatomic causes of bleeding including uterine fibroids, cervical or vaginal lesions or infection, cervical & endometrial cancer

2) Evaluate stress, exercise, weight changes, systemic disease such as thyroid, renal or hepatic disease & coagulopathies, & pregnancy

f. Tx

1) Convert proliferative endometrium into secretory endometrium by administration of a progestational agent for 10 days

2) Alternative is to give OCPs that suppress the endometrium & establish regular, predictable cycles

3) NSAIDs ⊕ iron used in pts who want to preserve fertility

4) **Postmenopausal bleeding is cancer until proven otherwise**

3. Menopause

a. Defined as the cessation of menses, **average age in the US is 51 yr**

b. Suspect when menstrual cycles are not regular & predictable, & when cycles are not associated with any premenstrual symptoms

c. Si/Sx = rapid onset hot flashes & sweating with resolution in 3 min, mood changes, sleep disturbances, vaginal dryness/atrophy, dyspareunia (painful intercourse), & osteoporosis

d. Dx = irregular menstrual cycles, hot flashes & ↑ FSH level (>30 mIU/mL)

e. Depending on clinical scenario, other laboratory tests should be conducted to exclude other diagnoses that can cause amenorrhea, such as thyroid disease, hyperprolactinemia, pregnancy

f. Tx

1) **First line is estrogen hormone replacement therapy (HRT)**

2) HRT can be via continuous estrogen with cyclic progestin to allow controlled withdrawal bleeding, or via daily administration of both estrogen & progestin, which does not cause withdrawal bleeding

3) There are risks & benefits of HRT

4) Raloxifene

a) Second-generation tamoxifen-like drug = mixed estrogen agonist/antagonist, FDA approved to prevent osteoporosis

b) So far raloxifene shown to act like estrogen in bones (good), ↓ serum LDL (good) but does not stimulate endometrial growth (good) (unlike tamoxifen & estrogen alone), effects on breast are not yet known

5) **Calcium supplements are not a substitute for estrogen replacement**

4. Infertility

   a. Defined as failure to conceive after 1 yr of unprotected sex

   b. Affects 10–15% of reproductive-age couples in the US

   c. Causes = abnormal spermatogenesis (40%), anovulation (30%), anatomic defects of the female reproductive tract (20%), unknown (10%)

   d. Dx

      1) **Start work-up with male partner not only because it is the most common cause,** but because the work-up is simpler, noninvasive, & more cost-effective than work-up of infertility in the female

      2) **Normal semen excludes male cause in >90% of couples**

      3) Work-up of female partner should include measurement of basal body temperature, which is an excellent screening test for ovulation

         a) Temperature drops at time of menses, then rises 2 days after LH surge at the time of progesterone rise

         b) Ovulation probably occurs 1 day before first temperature elevation, & temperature remains elevated for 13–14 days

         c) A temperature elevation of >16 days suggests pregnancy

      4) Anovulation

         a) Hx of regular menses with premenstrual Sx (breast fullness, ↓ vaginal secretions, abdominal bloating, mood changes) strongly suggests ovulation

         b) Sx such as irregular menses, amenorrhea episodes, hirsutism, acne, galactorrhea, suggest anovulation

         c) FSH measured at day 2–3 is best predictor of fertility potential in women, FSH >25IU/L correlated with a poor prognosis

         d) Dx confirm with basal body temperature, serum progesterone (↑ postovulation, >10 ng/mL → ovulation), endometrial Bx

      5) Anatomic disorder

         a) **Most commonly results from an acquired disorder, especially acute salpingitis 2° to *N. gonorrhoeae* & *C. trachomatis***

      b) Endometriosis, scarring, adhesions from pelvic inflammation or previous surgeries, tumors & trauma can also disrupt normal reproductive tract anatomy

      c) Less commonly a congenital anomaly such as septate uterus or reduplication of the uterus, cervix, or vagina is responsible

      d) **Dx with hysterosalpingogram**

e. Tx

  1) Anovulation → restore ovulation with use of ovulation-inducing drugs

    a) First line = clomiphene, an estrogen antagonist that relieves negative feedback on FSH, allowing follicle development

    b) Anovulatory women who bleed in response to progesterone are candidates for clomiphene, as are women with irregular menses or midluteal progesterone levels <10 ng/mL

    c) Forty percent get pregnant, 8–10% ↑ rate of multiple births, mostly twins

    d) If no response, FSH can be given directly → pregnancy rates of 60–80%, multiple births occur at an ↑ rate of 20%

      1) Anatomic abnormalities → surgical lysis of pelvic adhesions

      2) If endosalpinx is not intact & transport of the ovum is not possible, an assisted fertilization technique, such as *in vitro* fertilization, may be used with 15–25% success

XVII. COMMON SPORTS MEDICINE COMPLAINTS

A. Low Back Pain

1. Eighty percent of people experience low back pain—second most common complaint in 1° care (next to common cold)

2. **Fifty percent of cases will recur within the subsequent 3 yr**

3. **Majority of cases attributed to muscle strains,** but always consider disk herniation

4. Si/Sx of disk herniation = shooting pain down leg (sciatica),

pain on **straight leg raise (>90% sensitive)** & pain on **crossed straight leg raise (>90% specific, not sensitive)**

5. Dx

   a. **Always rule out RED FLAGS** (see below) with Hx & physical exam

   b. If no red flags detected, presume Dx is muscle strain & not serious; **no radiologic testing is warranted**

   c. Dz not remitting after 4 wk of conservative Tx should be further evaluated with repeat Hx & physical; consider radiologic studies

   d. Red flags (Table 31)

6. Tx

   a. No red flags → conservative with acetaminophen (safer) or NSAIDs, **muscle relaxants have not been shown to help**; avoid narcotics

   b. **Strict bed rest is NOT warranted** (extended rest shown to be debilitating, especially in older patients)—encourage return to normal activity, low-stress aerobic, & back exercises

   c. **Ninety percent of cases resolve within 4 wk with conservative Tx**

   d. Red flags:

      1) Fracture → surgical consult

      2) Tumor → urgent radiation/steroid (↓ compression), then excise

      3) Infection → abscess drainage & antibiotics per pathogen

      4) Cauda equina syndrome → emergent surgical decompression

      5) Spinal stenosis → complete laminectomy

      6) Radiculopathy → anti-inflammatories, nerve root decompression with laminectomy or microdiscectomy only if (1) sciatica is severe & disabling, (2) Sx persist for 4 wk or worsening progression, & (3) strong evidence of specific nerve root damage with MRI correlation of level of disk herniation

B. Shoulder Dislocation

1. Subluxation = symptomatic translation of humeral head relative to glenoid articular surface

TABLE 31	Low Back Pain Red Flags	
DIAGNOSIS	**Si/Sx**	**Dx**
Fracture	• Hx of trauma (fall, car accident) • Minor trauma in elderly (e.g., strenuous lifting)	• Spine x-rays
Tumor	• **Pt >50 yr old** (accounts for >80% of cancer cases) or <20 yr old • Prior Hx of CA • **Constitutional Sx** (fever/chills, weight loss) • Pain worse when supine or at night	• Spinal MRI is gold standard, can get CT also
Infection	• Immunosuppressed pts • Constitutional Sx • Recent bacterial infection or IV drug abuse	• Blood cultures, spinal MRI to rule out abscess
Cauda equina syndrome	• Acute urinary retention, **saddle anesthesia**, lower extremity weakness or paresthesias & ↓ reflexes, ↓ anal sphincter tone	• Spinal MRI
Spinal stenosis	• Si/Sx = **pseudoclaudication** (neurogenic) with pain ↑ with walking **& standing**; relieved by sitting or leaning forward	• Spinal MRI
Radiculopathy (herniation compressing spinal nerves)*	• Sensory loss: (**L5** →Large toe/medial foot, **S1**→ Small toe/lateral foot) • Weakness: (L1–L4 →quadriceps, L5 → foot dorsiflexion, S1 → plantar flexion) • ↓ reflexes (L4 →patellar, S1 →achilles)	• **Clinical**—MRI may confirm clinical Dx but false-positive are common (clinically insignificant disk herniation)

*Radiculopathy ≠ herniation; radiculopathy indicates evolving spinal nerve impingement & is a more serious Dx than simple herniation indicated by straight leg testing & sciatica.

2. Dislocation = complete displacement out of the glenoid

3. Anterior instability (about 95% of cases) usually due to subcoracoid dislocation is the most common form of shoulder dislocation

4. Si/Sx = pain, joint immobility, arm "goes dead" with overhead motion

5. Dx = clinical, assess axillary nerve function in neuro exam, look for signs of rotator cuff injury, confirm with x-rays if necessary

6. Tx = initial reduction of dislocation by various traction-countertraction techniques, 2–6 wk period of immobilization (longer for younger patients), intense rehabilitation; rarely is surgery required

C. Clavicle Fracture

1. Occurs primarily due to contact sports in adults

2. Si/Sx = pain & deformity at clavicle

3. Dx = clinical, confirm fracture with standard AP view x-ray

4. Must rule out subclavian artery injury by checking pulses, brachial plexus injury with neuro examination, and pneumothorax by checking breath sounds

5. Tx = sling until range of motion is painless (usually 2–4 wk)

D. Elbow Injuries

1. Epicondylitis (tendinitis)

   a. Lateral epicondylitis (**tennis elbow**)

      1) Usually in tennis player (>50%), or racquetball, squash, fencing

      2) Si/Sx = pain 2–5 cm distal & anterior to lateral epicondyle reproduced with wrist extension while elbow is extended

   b. Medial epicondylitis (**golfer's elbow**)

      1) Commonly in golf, racquet sports, bowling, baseball, swimming

      2) Si/Sx = acute onset of medial elbow pain & swelling

          localized 1 or 2 cm area distal to medial epicondyle, pain usually reproduced with wrist flexion, & pronation against resistance

   c. Tx for both = ice, rest, NSAIDs, counterforce bracing, rehabilitation

   d. Px for both varies, can become chronic condition; surgery sometimes indicated (débridement & tendon reapproximation)

2. Olecranon fracture

   a. Usually direct blow to elbow with triceps contraction after fall on flexed upper extremity

   b. Tx = long arm cast or splint in 45–90° flexion for ≥3 wk

   c. Displaced fracture requires open reduction & internal fixation

3. Dislocation

   a. Elbow joint most commonly dislocated joint in children, second most in adults (next to shoulder)

   b. Fall onto outstretched hand with fully extended elbow (posterolateral dislocation) or direct blow to posterior elbow (anterior dislocation)

   c. May also be seen after jerking child's arm by hurried parent or guardian (**nurse-maid's elbow**)

   d. Key is associated nerve injury (ulnar, median, radial or anterior interosseous nerve), vascular injury (brachial artery) or other structural injury (associated coronoid process fracture common)

   e. Tx = reduce elbow by gently flexing supinated arm, long arm splint or bivalved cast applied at 90° flexion

4. Olecranon bursitis

   a. Inflammation of bursa under olecranon process

   b. Seen with direct blow to elbow by collision or fall on artificial turf

   c. Si/Sx = swollen & painful posterior elbow with restricted motion

   d. Dx = clinical, confirm with bursa aspiration to rule out septic bursitis

e. Tx = bursa aspiration, compression dressing & pad

E. Ankle Injuries

1. Achilles tendonitis

   a. 2° to overuse, commonly seen in runners, gymnasts, cyclists, & volleyball players

   b. Si/Sx = swelling or erythema along area of Achilles tendon with tenderness 2–5 cm proximal to calcaneus

   c. Evaluate for rupture = Thompson test (squeezing leg with passive plantar flexion) positive only with complete tear

   d. Tx = rest, ice, NSAIDs, taping or splinting to $\downarrow$ stress & $\uparrow$ support

   e. Rupture requires long leg casting × 4 wk, short leg walking cast × 4 wk, then wear heel lift × 4 wk

   f. Open repair speeds recovery & is recommended with complete tears in younger patients

2. Ankle sprains

   a. Lateral sprain occurs when ankle is plantar-flexed (90% of sprains)

   b. Anterior drawer sign is done with foot in 10–15° plantar flexion

   c. Medial sprain is rare (10%) because ligament is stronger

   d. Dx = multiple view x-rays both free & weight bearing

   e. Tx = **RICE** = **R**est (limit activity +/– crutches), **I**ce, **C**ompression (ACE bandage), **E**levation above level of heart to decrease swelling

   e. Severe sprains may benefit from casting, open repair rarely indicated

XVIII. PREVENTIVE MEDICINE

A. Cancer Screening (Table 32)

TABLE 32	Cancer Screening
DISEASE	**INTERVENTION**
Cervical CA	• Annual PS in women ≥18 yr or sexually active (ACS) • Perform less often if ≥3 consecutive Paps are nl & pt is monogamous
Breast CA	• Exam & mammogram every 1–2 yr in women 50–69 yr (AAFP, USPTF) • Self exams; annual exam & mammogram in women >40 yr (ACS)
Colorectal CA	• Hemoccult annually >50 yr (screen earlier with positive family Hx) • Pt >50 yr → sigmoidoscopy q 5 yr or colonoscopy q 10 yr (ACS)
Prostate CA	• Annual digital exam & PSA should be offered to all men >50 yr (ACS)
Endometrial CA	• High-risk patients should have biopsy shortly after menopause (ACS)
Other CA	• Annual physical exam for signs of thyroid, skin, oral, testicular or ovarian CA (ACS)

B. Adult Immunization (Table 33)

TABLE 33	Adult Immunization
Tetanus	All require primary series & periodic boosters q 10 yr (A)
MMR	All require vaccination if born after 1956 without immunity (A)
Hepatitis B	Recommended for all young adults & ↑ risk pts (A)
Pneumo-coccal	Give once in immunocompetent pts ≥65 yr or to any pt with ↑ risk (B)
Influenza	Annually for all pts ≥50* yr or high-risk pts (B)
Hepatitis A	Only for high-risk patients like travelers (B)
Varicella	Adults without Hx of disease or previous vaccination (B) In HIV pts avoid live preparations, but MMR should be given if CD4 count >500 In pregnant pts, live vaccinations are not recommended (MMR, OPV, VZV)
A = proven benefit, B = probably benefit. * New rec in 2000.	

C. Travel Prophylaxis (Table 34)

TABLE 34	Travel Prophylaxis
Traveler's Diarrhea	Prevent w/Pepto-Bismol; Tx w/ciprofloxacin & loperamide
Malaria	Chloroquine; mefloquine (endemic chloroquine-resistant areas)
Hepatitis A	Most travelers; vaccine requires 4 wk; give IVIG for short-term
Typhoid	Endemic in India, Pakistan, Peru, Chile, Mexico; oral or inject
Yellow fever	Endemic in parts of South America & Africa
Meningococcus	Endemic in meningococcal belt (sub-Saharan Africa) Ensure all other routine immunizations are up to date (MMR, polio, Hep B)

Note: Current cholera & plague vaccines are not very effective.

D. Smoking Cessation

1. Twenty to fifty million US smokers attempt to quit; 6% long-term success rate

2. **Nicotine replacement (gum or patch) increases success about two-fold**

3. Support from weekly counseling sessions, telephone calls, family & other support groups shown ↑ success

4. For best success, set a precise quit date to begin complete abstinence

5. Pts with negative affect (e.g., depression) have more difficulty quitting

6. **Bupropion +/– nicotine replacement** has 12 mo abstinence rate of >30%, **2x better than nicotine replacement alone** [*New Engl J Med* 1999, 340:9, 655]

7. On average, pts who quit successfully will gain weight (mean = 5 lb)

E. Other Periodic Health Examination Concerns

1. Adolescence (11–24 yr)

   a. Leading cause of death are MVA, & injuries, & homicide/suicide

TABLE 35	Tetanus Immunization		
IMMUNIZATION HISTORY	**NON TETANUS PRONE WOUNDS**	**TETANUS PRONE WOUNDS**
Unknown schedule or less than three injections	Td	Tetanus Immune Globulin(TIG) + Td
Last Injection <10 yr ago	None	Td
Last Injection >10 yr ago	Td	Td

   b. BP check, Pap smears, rubella status, drug & STD education, safety

2. HTN: check BP every 2 yr in normotensive pts 21+yr

3. Hyperlipidemia: check cholesterol & lipids in normal population about every 5 yr in men 35–65 yr, & women 45–65 yr

4. Endocarditis: antibiotic prophylaxis (amoxicillin or erythromycin) given before & after dental procedures & certain surgeries; consider prophylaxis for (1) prosthetic values, (2) mitral or aortic valvular dz, (3) congenital heart dz, & (4) prior Hx of infectious endocarditis. Check with cardiologist for latest recommendations

5. Tetanus immunization: Tetanus prone wounds >6 hr old, contaminated, puncture, crush, missile, burn, or frostbite (Table 35)

XIX. LAW AND ETHICS

A. Legal Issues

1. Malpractice

   a. A civil wrong doing (tort), not a crime

   b. Must satisfy the four "Ds"

      1) Dereliction: deviation from the applicable standard of care

      2) Duty: a physician–patient relationship was established with a duty to treat

3) Damages: injury or measurable damages occur

4) Directly: injury or damages directly result from physicians actions or inactions

c. May be required to pay compensatory damages (money) for patient's suffering

d. Studies have shown physicians with poor communication skills and interactions with patients are most likely to be sued for malpractice

2. Informed consent

a. Must be obtained from patient by a physician knowledgeable in the diagnosis and treatment in question before any procedure

b. Patients must be presented with their diagnosis, potential treatments, and the risks and benefits of each treatment

c. A competent adult or emancipated minor must then voluntarily consent or not consent to the treatment prior to starting

d. Considered *Battery* or *Negligence* if not obtained

e. In an emergency, if patient is unable to consent, life-saving measures may be provided

3. Confidentiality

a. Fosters trust in doctor–patient relationship and respects patient's privacy

b. Can be overridden if there is a potential harm to a third party and there is no less invasive way for warning or protecting those at risk

4. *Primum non nocer*, Nonmaleficence

a. "Above all do no harm"

b. A balance must exist in the care of patients. Risks and benefits of all interventions must be considered

c. If a physician can't act to benefit the patient, then at least do no harm

5. Beneficence

a. Fiduciary relationship exists between the doctor and patient

b. Physicians are trusted to act on behalf of the well being of their patients

6. Death

   a. With the advent of cardiopulmonary life support systems the definition of death is no longer simply a cessation of breathing or circulation

   b. Death is now also defined as complete irreversible loss of entire brain function to include cortical and brain stem function

   c. Patients must be "warm and dead" to be considered dead, there are many stories of people revived from freezing cold temperatures who where thought to be dead

   d. Persistent Vegetative State (PVS): have brain stem function but no cortical function

7. Advance directives

   a. Allows competent patients to indicate their health-related preferences or a surrogate decision-maker prior to becoming incapacitated

   b. Living Will: Written instructions related to health-related preferences in the event the patient becomes incapacitated and is unable to communicate his or her wishes otherwise

   c. Durable Power of Attorney: A surrogate is designated to make health care decisions on behalf of the incapacitated patient

   d. Various states have limitations on Advance Directives; an attorney should be consulted if there are any questions regarding your particular state

8. Do Not Resuscitate orders (DNR)

   a. Can only be initiated by the attending staff physician after receiving informed consent from appropriate health care decision-maker

   b. Cardiopulmonary Resuscitation (CPR) is withheld

   c. Limited DNR orders may also be seen such as DNI (Do not Intubate), and chest compressions only

   d. These should all be clearly visible to all staff so that patient's requests can be followed in an emergency

XX. BIOSTATISTICS

A. Table of Definitions (Table 36)

TABLE 36	Biostatistics and Epidemiology
TERM	**DEFINITION**
Sensitivity	Probability that test results will be positive in pts with disease
Specificity	Probability that test results will be negative in pts without disease
False-positive	Pt without disease who has a positive test result
False-negative	Pt with disease who has a negative test result
PPV	Positive predictive value: probability pt with positive test actually has disease
NPV	Negative predictive value: probability pt with negative test actually has no disease
Incidence	No. of newly reported cases of disease, divided by total population
Prevalence	No. of existing cases of disease, divided by total population at a given time
Relative risk	From cohort study (prospective)—risk of developing dz for people with known exposure, compared to risk of developing dz without exposure
Attributable risk	The difference between incidence rates of the exposed and nonexposed
Odds ratio	From case control study (retrospective)—approximates relative risk by comparing odds of developing dz in exposed pts to odds of developing dz in unexposed pts (if dz is rare, odds ratio approaches true relative risk)
Variance	An estimate of the variability of each individual data point from the mean
STD deviation	Square root of the variance
Type I error (α error)	Null hypothesis is rejected even though it is true, e.g., the study says the intervention works but it only appears to work because of random chance
Type II error (β error)	Null hypothesis is not rejected even though it is false, e.g., the study fails to detect a true effect of the intervention
Power ($1 - \beta$)	An estimate of the probability a study will be able to detect a true effect of the intervention, e.g., power of 80% means that if the intervention works, the study has an 80% chance of detecting this but a 20% chance of randomly missing it

B. Study Types

Prospective is more powerful than retrospective. Interventional is more powerful than observational

1. Clinical trial: **Prospective interventional trial,** in which pts are randomized into an intervention group & a control group. **Randomization blunts effect of confounding factors. Blinding both clinician & patient (double-blind) further decreases bias**

2. Cohort study: Population is divided by exposure status. Requires large population (cannot study rare disease). Can study multiple effects by exposure. Gives **relative risk if prospective.** Can be prospective or retrospective

3. Case control study: Pts divided by those with dz (cases) and those without dz (controls). Fewer patients are needed (good for rare disease). Can study correlation of multiple exposures. Gives **odds ratio. Always retrospective**

C. Calculation of Statistical Values

Sensitivity & specificity are inherent characteristics of the test; they must be given in the question. **Predictive values vary with the prevalence of the disease.** They are NOT inherent characteristics of the test, but rather reflect an interaction of sensitivity & specificity with the frequency of the disease in the population

EXAMPLE 1	For disease X, a theoretical screening test is **90% sensitive & 80% specific.** In Africa, where the disease has a **prevalence of 50%,** the test's **PPV = 82%** (a/a + b = 45/55), & the **NPV is 89%** (d/c + d = 40/45).

	PT HAS DZ	PT DOES NOT HAVE DZ
Positive test	45	10
Negative test	5	40

Note: PPV = Positive Predictive Value; NPV = Negative Predictive Value.

Always fill the table in assuming 100 patients: it's easier to do the math this way. The prevalence of the disease (50%) tells you that 50 patients should be in the first column, because 50% of 100 patients have the disease. Therefore, 50 patients should also be in the second column (if 50 of 100 patients have the disease, 50 patients also do NOT have the disease). The sensitivity tells you that

45 of the patients in the first column should be in the top row because the test will find 90% of the 50 patients who have the disease. The specificity tells you that 40 of the patients in the second column should be in the bottom row because the test will correctly describe 80% of the 50 people who truly don't have the disease (& incorrectly claim that 20% of the 50 patients who truly don't have the disease do have the disease).

EXAMPLE 2	Now study the **same test for the same disease (X)** in America, where the **prevalence of the disease is 10%**. The test characteristics remain the same: **90% sensitive & 80% specific**. The test's **PPV = 33%** (a/a + b = 9/27) & the **NPV = 99%** (d/c + d = 72/73). **The same test has drastically different values depending on the disease prevalence!**

	PT HAS DZ	PT DOES NOT HAVE DZ
Positive test	9	18
Negative test	1	72

Now the disease prevalence tells you that 10 patients should be in the first column (10% of 100 patients have the disease). Therefore, 90 patients should be in the second column (if 10 of 100 patients have the disease, 90 patients do NOT have the disease). The sensitivity tells you that 9 of the patients in the first column should be in the top row because the test will find 90% of the 10 patients who have the disease. The specificity tells you that 72 of the patients in the second column should be in the bottom row because the test will correctly describe 80% of the 90 people who truly don't have the disease (& incorrectly claim that 20% of the 90 patients who don't have the disease do have the disease).

TABLE 37	Sample Calculation of Statistical Values		
	PT HAS DZ	PT DOES NOT HAVE DZ	PPV = a/a + b
Positive test	a = true-positive	b = false-positive	NPV = d/c + d
Negative test	c = false-negative	d = true-negative	Sensitivity = a/a + c
			Specificity = d/b + d

REVIEW QUESTIONS

1. A 25-yr-old female presents to your urgent care clinic with her 4-yr-old son. The mother tells you that her little boy has just fallen in the playground. You examine the child and notice that he has bruises that are bilateral, symmetric, and

different colors. The bruises are on the back of his hands, buttocks, and back. You then take a better look at the mother and notice that she has her left arm in a cast. What do you do next to help this family?

a) You explain to her not to worry about her child's injuries because they are minor and will quickly heal

b) You ask to further examine the mother for the possibility of other broken bones

c) You explain to the mother that you suspect abuse in the family and that you are required by law to call children's protective services. You also advise her that there are shelters for battered women that can assist this family with a safe place to stay, and a social worker will soon be here to discuss her options

d) You allow her to leave after you have treated her child and then you look on the urgent care check-in sheet for her address and call the police to investigate her house for suspected child abuse

2. A 16-yr-old female is brought into your pediatric clinic by her mother who thinks the daughter is pregnant. After a long discussion, in which the mother explains how hard she has worked to properly raise this child, the mother tells you that her daughter has not had her menses in the past two months, throws up every morning, constantly c/o constipation, and is constantly wearing big sweaters to hide her belly. You ask your nurse to come in the room and explain to the mother that you must question her daughter privately first. The mother agrees and then you do which of the following?

a) Immediately ask the 16-yr-old female to tell you what this is all about and stop wasting your time

b) Inform her that whatever she tells you is confidential except if suicide, homicide, or abuse is concerned

c) Perform your exam and then immediately call in the mother and review your findings

d) Examine the mother for possible referral to a teen-daughter support group

3. After interviewing and examining the 16-yr-old female, you check labs and an EKG and note the following findings: emaciation, cardiac arrhythmia, tooth decay, anemia, and fluid & electrolyte abnormalities. You also verify her sexual hx, obtain a negative, urine HCG, verify the history of ammenorhea and then ask her about her diet hx. You then

inform both of them of the following potential diagnosis and treatment:

a) The 16 yr old is pregnant and possibly it is too early to detect with a urine pregnancy test. It is obvious she is suffering from morning sickness. You give them iron supplements and antiemetics that will not harm the fetus.

b) This teenager probably has bulimia, as evidenced by poor dentition, vomiting, and poor body image. She will be referred to a child psychiatrist or psychologist for treatment after a short hospitalization to correct her electrolyte abnormalities.

c) This teenager has no problems and the mother should be referred to a teen-daughter support group.

d) This 16-yr-old girl has all the classic findings of Anorexia nervosa. She may need to be admitted to the hospital to correct her electrolyte abnormalities and to observe her eating habits. You will discuss this with the child psychiatrist.

4. Match the following signs and symptoms with the possible intoxicating substance. Each choice will be used only once:

1) Hypotension and bradycardia   a) Ciguatera Toxin

2) Tachycardia, hypertension weight loss   b) Organophosphates

3) GI Complaints after eating Barracuda   c) Scombroid

4) Rigid abdominal muscles, vomiting, pain in extremity   d) Opiods

5) Flushed face, burning sensation in mouth after eating marine tuna   e) Lead poisoning

6) Microcytic anemia with basophilic stippling purple lines on teeth   f) Black widow spider

7) Decreased consciousness, pinpoint pupils respiratory depression   g) Ma huang

5. Match the following signs and symptoms with the psychiatric diagnosis:

1) Depressive episodes with hypo-manic episodes, no manic episodes   a) Dysthymic disorder

2) Hallucinations, lack of affect, disorganized behavior lasting less than 6 mo   b) Bipolar II

3) Continuous depressive symptoms for at least 2 yr

   c) Schizoid

4) Socially withdrawn, recognizes reality, blunt affect

   d) Trichotillomania

5) Hair pulling resulting in observable hair loss

   e) Schitzophreniform

6. A 40-yr-old male comes into your community clinic and the nurse asks him to wait in your examining room. When you walk in you notice a large, obese man asleep in your examining chair, snoring loudly. You attempt to wake him but it proves to be very difficult. When he finally wakes up he tells you another doctor checked his blood and found his hematocrit to be elevated. The other doctor then advised him to have surgery to correct his snoring. What do you think this patient may have and is surgery indicated?

   a) This patient obviously has narcolepsy as evidenced by his recurrent sleep attacks

   b) He has central obstructive sleep apnea that can only be treated with surgery

   c) This patient has the classic triad of Pickwickian Syndrome and the first-line treatment is weight loss

   d) This patient has no need to have surgery or lose weight, a CPAP machine at night will solve his problems

7. A 78-yr-old Chinese male comes into your office alone. He speaks only Mandarin and he is trying to explain to you something related to his knees and elbows. You graciously greet him and ask him to wait for the interpreter to arrive. Once the interpreter arrives, he explains to her that for twenty years he has used needles and herbs to treat his joint pains. He has heard of certain new medications that may be of some use and would like information. You then begin talking directly to the Mandarin interpreter and inform her of the anti-inflammatory cyclo-oxygenase inhibitors. You tell the translator that the patient should also have a prostate exam, PSA test, and sigmoidoscopy prior to starting these meds since he is over 50 years old. After a lengthy discussion with the translator, you finally allow her to translate your entire set of recommendations. Upon hearing the translation, the patient begins shouting. The translator tells you the patient is upset because you insulted him by offering to examine his colon when all he wanted was arthritis medicine. How could this incident have been avoided?

a) Next time act out with your hands what you are describing to the translator so that the patient, if he is looking, can visualize the instructions

b) Next time face the patient, and explain all instructions carefully to him, allowing the translator time to translate by pausing frequently. Then ask the patient during the interview if he has any questions. Finally, ask the patient to repeat your instructions to assure that he fully understands

c) Next time, don't call for an interpreter and just prescribe strong narcotic medications for his pain

d) Next time, have the patient bring a family member to translate for him

8. Match the following terms with their corresponding definitions:

1) Sensitivity	a) Difference between incidence rates of the exposed and non-exposed
2) Prevalence	b) Probability that a test result will be negative in patients without disease
3) Variance	c) Probability that a test result will be positive in patients with disease
4) Attributable risk	d) The number of existing cases of a disease divided by the total population at a given time
5) Specificity	e) An estimate of the variability of each individual data point from the mean
6) Nonmalficence	f) Trusted to act on behalf of the well being of patients
7) Beneficence	g) Above all do no harm

ANSWERS

1. **c)** The law requires that all suspected cases of child abuse must be reported to child protective services. Depending on

the state you practice in, spouse abuse may also require reporting. People who suffer from this type of abuse frequently hospital-shop so hospital personnel will not recognize the pattern of abuse. Therefore it is very unlikely that they will give any factual information during their check in.

2. **b)** In order to establish trust you must first assure the adolescent that your conversation is confidential. This is especially important in areas concerning sex or drugs. By removing the mom from the room you can establish this trust and therefore gain more information to assist the patient and the family. The mom may still need a support group to deal with her daughter's possible diagnosis.

3. **d)** The classic symptoms of ammenorrhea, weight loss >15%, constipation, electrolyte and cardiac abnormalities are all present in this female. This dangerous combination can be fatal. Therefore hospitalization is indicated to better observe the patient and correct her electrolyte imbalance. Bulimic patients generally appear healthier and also have poor dentition from frequent self-induced vomiting episodes.

4. **1-b, 2-g, 3-a, 4-f, 5-c, 6-e, 7-d.**

5. **1-b, 2-e, 3-a, 4-c, 5-d.**

6. **c)** Pickwickian Syndrome describes the triad of somnolence, obesity, and erythrocytosis. Treatment is weight loss. There is no such thing as a central obstructive disorder. Central sleep apnea is related to lack of respiratory drive, whereas obstructive sleep apnea is related to mechanical blockade of ventilation. Patients with narcolepsy have sudden uncontrolled drop attacks unlike our patient.

7. **b)** Effective patient doctor communication requires sufficient time. An interpreter should be available to assist with communication. Family members and friends should not be used unless absolutely necessary. This places the patient in embarrassing situations and does not assure that what you are saying is fully understood by the person translating. You should always speak directly to the patient and ask questions frequently to avoid any misunderstandings.

8. **1-c, 2-d, 3-e, 4-a, 5-b, 6-g, 7-f.**

INDEX

A

Abstract thoughts, 7t
Abuse. *See also* Child abuse
    identifying, 3–4
    mandatory reporting of, 3
Acetaminophen, 42t
Achievement tests, 9t
Achilles tendonitis, 75
Acquired immunodeficiency
    syndrome
        course of, 58–59
        etiology of, 55–57
        HIV biology in, 57–58
        treatment of, 59
Acting out, 30
Activities, patient, 2
Acyclovir
    for herpes simplex virus, 56t
    for otitis externa, 49
Adenomyosis, 65
Adenovirus, 50t
Adjustment disorder, 34
Adolescence
    confidentiality and, 14
    eating disorders of, 14
    health examination during, 77–78
    injuries in, 13
    pregnancy during, 84, 88
    psychiatric disorders during, 14–18
    sexual activity in, 14
    substance abuse in, 13–14
    suicide in, 13
Advance directives, 80
Agoraphobia, 26t
AIDS. *See* Acquired immunodeficiency
    syndrome
Akathisia, antipsychotic-associated, 25t
Albumin serum levels, 38
Alcohol abuse, 19t
Alkali agents, 42t
Alpha waves, 36t
Alternative medical practices, 85, 88
    incorporation of, 38, 88
Amenorrhea, 62, 66–67
    anorexia nervosa in, 84–85, 88
Amitriptyline
    for depression, 22t
    for posttraumatic stress
        disorder, 27t
Amnesia, dissociative, 33
Amphetamine
    abuse of, 19t
    for attention-deficit hyperactivity
        disorder, 16
Amyl nitrite, 42t

Animal bites, 45–46t
Ankle
    injuries of, 75
    sprained, 75
Anorexia nervosa, 17
    in adolescents, 14
    signs of, 84–85, 88
Anovulation, 67, 69
    treatment of, 70
Antacids, 51
Anthropometric measurements, 38
Anti-digoxin, 42t
Anticholinergic drugs, 42t
Antidepressants, 22t
    for pediatric depression, 15
    for posttraumatic stress
        disorder, 27t
    for tension headache, 48t
Antiemetics, 48t
Antipsychotic drugs, 24t
    movement disorders associated
        with, 25t
Antisocial personality, characteristics
    of, 29t
Antivenin
    for black widow spider bite, 45t
    for snake bite, 46t
Anxiety, 26–27t
    in impulsive-control disorders, 34
Arsenic, 42t
Asherman's syndrome, 66
Asperger's syndrome, 14
Aspirin, 42t
Atropine, 43t
Attention-deficit hyperactivity disorder
    (ADHD), 16
Attributable risk, 81t, 87–88, 88
Autism, 14
Autoimmune ovarian failure, 67
Avoidant personality, 30t
Azithromycin (AZT), 59

B

Bacterial vaginosis, 64
Bacteriuria, asymptomatic, 55
Bactrim
    for infectious diarrhea, 55t
    for urinary tract infection, 55
Barbiturate abuse, 19t
Barrett's esophagus, 52
Basal body temperature, 69
Bee sting, 45t
Behavioral therapy
    for impotence, 62
    for psychotic disorders, 24

Beneficence, 79
definition of, 87–88
Benign prostatic hyperplasia, 60–61
Benzathine penicillin G, 57t
Benzodiazepine
for delirium, 35t
for panic disorder, 26t
signs and symptoms of abuse, 19t
toxicology and antidotes of, 42t
Bereavement, 34
signs and symptoms of, 21t
Beriberi, 40t
β-blockers
for agoraphobia, 26t
for generalized anxiety
disorder, 27t
for migraine, 48t
for tension headache, 48t
toxicology and antidotes of, 42t
Bicarbonate
for aspirin poisoning, 42t
for methanol poisoning, 43t
for phenobarbitol poisoning, 43t
for tricyclic poisoning, 43t
Bilzzard's syndrome, 67
Biofeedback, 27t
Biostatistics, 80–83
Biotin, deficiencies and excesses of, 40t
Bipolar disorder, 21t
Bites, 45–46t
Bitot's spots, 41t
Black widow spider bite, 45t
Blood dyscrasia, 22
Body dysmorphic disorder, 32–33
Body mass index (BMI), 38
Borderline personality, 29t
Breast cancer screening, 76t
Brevitoxin, 45t
Bronze diabetes, 40t
Brown recluse spider bite, 46t
Bulimia, 18
in adolescents, 14
Bupropion, 77
Burns, 11
Bursitis, olecranon, 74–75
Buspirone, 27t

C

Caida de la mollera, 4
Calcium, 42t
Calcium-channel blockers, 22
Caloric requirements, 39
Calories, deficiencies and excesses
of, 41t
Cancer screening, 76t
Candida infection, pharyngeal, 50t
Candida vaginitis, 64
differential diagnosis of, 65t

Capitation, 5
Carbamazepine
for mania, 22
for temporal arteritis, 48t
Carbon monoxide, 42t
Cardiac monitor, 43t
Cardiopulmonary life support
systems, 80
Cardiopulmonary resuscitation (CPR), 80
Case control study, 82
Cat bite, 46t
Cauda equina syndrome, 71
in low back pain, 71, 72t
CD4 T cells, in AIDS, 58–59
Celiac sprue, 53t
Central alveolar hypoventilation, 37
Cephalosporin, 56t
Cervical cancer screening, 76t
Charcoal
for child poisonings, 12
for phenobarbitol poisoning, 43t
for theophylline poisoning, 43t
Cheilosis, 40t
Chief complaint, 1
Child abuse, 10–12
classic findings of, 10–11
epidemiology of, 10
examination for and reporting of,
83–84, 87–88
Children
confidentiality with, 14
psychiatric disorders in, 14–18
trauma and intoxication in, 10–12
Chip fracture, 10
Chlamydia
in adolescents, 14
trachomatis, 56t
Chlorpromazine, 24t
Chromium, deficiencies and excesses
of, 40t
Cigarette burns, 11
Ciguatera toxin, 44t
Ciguatoxin, 44t
Ciprofloxacin, 53t, 55t
Clavicle fracture, 73
Clinical Nurse Specialist, 6
Clinical trial, 82
Clomipramine
for obsessive compulsive
disorder, 26t
for panic disorder, 26t
Clonazepam, 48t
Clotting deficiency, 41t
Clozapine, 24t
Cluster A personality, 28
Cluster B personality, 28
Cluster C personality, 28

Cluster headache
  epidemiology and characteristics
    of, 47t
  treatment of, 48t
Cocaine abuse, 19t
Cognition, developmental milestones
  of, 8t
Cognitive behavior, 27t
Cognitive-behavioral therapy, 26t
Cohort study, 82
Colorectal cancer screening, 76t
Colposcopy, 64
Communications, interpreter for, 4–5,
  85–86, 88
Community hospital, 5
Compensation claims, 31
Conduct disorder, 16
Cone biopsy, 64
Confidentiality, 79
  of adolescent pregnancy, 84, 88
  with children and adolescents, 14
Consent, informed, 79
Contraception, 63
Conversion disorder, 32
Copper, deficiencies and excesses of, 40t
Counseling, impotence, 62
Coxsackie A infection, 50t
Cultural demographics, 3
Cultural diversity, 1
Cultural medicine, 4, 88
Cultural medicine rituals, 3–4
Cupping, 3
Curandero, 4
Cyanide poisoning, 42t
Cyanocobalamin, deficiencies and
  excesses of, 40t
Cystic fibrosis, 54t
Cystoscopy, 60

D

Danazol, 65
Death, legal definition of, 80
Deferoxamine, 43t
Delirium
  versus dementia, 35t
  diagnosis of, 23t
Delta wave sleep, 36t
Delusional disorder, 23t
Delusions, 23
Dementia, 35t
Dependent personality, 30t
Depression
  in children and adolescents, 15
  diagnosis of, 23t
  treatment of, 21–22
Dereliction, 78
Dermatitis, 40t
Desensitization

  for agoraphobia, 26t
  for posttraumatic stress
    disorder, 27t
Desensitizing therapy, 16
Desipramine, 22t
Developmental milestones, 8t
Developmental theories, 7t
Diabetes insipidus, nephrogenic, 22
Diagnostic and Statistical Manual
  (DSM-IV) classification, 19
Dialysis, 42t
Diarrhea, 52
  infectious causes of, 55t
  traveler's, prophylaxis for, 77t
  types of, 53–54t
Diet history, 37
Digoxin, 42t
Dihydroergotamine
  for cluster headache, 48t
  for migraine, 48t
Dimercaprol
  for arsenic poisoning, 42t
  for mercury poisoning, 43t
Diphenhydramine, 45t
Diphtheria, 50t
Disassociative disorder, 33
Disk herniation, 70
Dislocation
  of elbow, 74
  shoulder, 71–73
Dissociative fugue, 33
Do not intubate (DNI), 80
Do not resuscitate orders (DNR), 80
Doctoral Nurses, 7
Doctoring, techniques of, 1–3
Dog bite, 46t
Dopamine-blockers, 24
Doxycycline, 56t
Drug abuse
  adolescent, 13–14
  agents of, 19
Drug-induced mania, 21t
Drug-induced psychosis, 23t
Drug use, patient history of, 2
Durable power of attorney, 80
Dysfunctional uterine bleeding, 67–68
Dysnomnias, 36–37
Dyspepsia, 50–51
Dysthymic disorder, 21t
Dystonia, antipsychotic-associated, 25t

E

Ear, nose, and throat complaints, 48–50
Eating disorders, 14. See also Anorexia
  nervosa; Bulimia
EDTA, 43t
Ego defenses, 28–30
Ego-dystonic behavior, 28

Ego-syntonic behavior, 28
Elbow injuries, 73–74
Electroconvulsive therapy, 22
Empacho, 4
Empathy, 2t
Employment & Education, 2
Encopresis, 53t
Endocarditis, 78
Endocervical curettage, 64
Endometrial cancer screening, 76t
Endometrioma, 65
Endometriosis, 64–66
  in infertility, 70
Enteral feeding, 39
Enteritis, 40t
Epicondylitis, 73–74
Epidemiology, terminology of, 81t
Epinephrine, 45t
Epistaxis, 49
Erectile dysfunction, 61
Ergotamine, 48t
Erickson developmental theory, 7t
Erythromycin, 46t
Escherichia coli, urinary tract, 55
Estradiol, 62
Estrogen deficiency, 66–67
Estrogen/progesterone
  contraceptives, 63
Estrogen/progestin contraceptives, 63
Estrogen replacement therapy
  for endometriosis, 66
  for menopause, 68
Ethanol drip
  for ethylene glycol poisoning, 42t
  for methanol poisoning, 43t
Ethylene glycol, 42t
Exposure desensitization
  for agoraphobia, 26t
  for posttraumatic stress
    disorder, 27t
Extended care facilities, 5–6
Exudative diarrhea, 53t

F

Fab-antibodies, 42t
Factitious disorders, 30–31
False-negative, 81t
False-positive, 81t
Famciclovir, 56t
Family history (FH), 1
Family therapy
  for pediatric depression, 15
  for psychotic disorders, 24
Female genital mutilation, 4
Fiber, dietary, 53t
Finasteride, 60
Fine motor developments, milestones
  of, 8t

Fire-setting, 34
Fish toxins, 44–45t
Fluconazole, 65t
Flumazenil, 42t
Fluoroquinolone
  for pelvic inflammatory disease, 56t
  for urinary tract infection, 55
Fluoxetine, 22t
Folate, 54t
Folic acid, deficiencies and excesses
  of, 40t
Folk healers, 4
Folk illness, 4
Folk medicine, incorporation of, 88
Follicle-stimulating hormone, 62, 69
Fomepizol, 42t
Foreign language patients, 4–5,
  85–86, 88
Fractures
  in child abuse, 10–11
  of clavicle, 73
  dating, 11
  in low back pain, 71, 72t
Fragile RBCs, 41t
Freudian developmental theory, 7t
Fugue, 33
Fundoplication, 52

G

Gardnerella vaginitis, 64, 65t
Gastric lavage, 42t
Gastroesophageal reflux disease (GERD),
  51–52
Gastrointestinal complaints, 50–52
Gender identity disorder, 33
Generalized anxiety disorder, 27t
Giant cell arteritis, 47t
Glucagon, 42t
Glucose intolerance, 40t
Golfer's elbow, 73–74
Gonadotropin-releasing hormone, 62
Gonadotropin-releasing hormone
  agonists, 65
Gonorrhea, 14
Gross motor developments,
  milestones of, 8t
Gynecological complaints, 62–66

H

H_2 blockers, 51
H_2-receptor antagonists, 51
Hair-pulling, 34
Hallucinations, 23
Haloperidol
  for delirium, 35t
  effects of, 24t
  for Tourette's disorder, 17
Harris-Benedict equation, 39
Head injury, 11

Headache
 diagnosis of, 47–48
 differential diagnosis of, 47t
 treatment of, 48t
HEADSSS mnemonic, 1–3
Health care delivery
 extended care facilities in, 5–6
 HMOs in, 5
 hospice in, 6
 hospital personnel in, 6–7
 hospitals in, 5
 Medicare/Medicaid in, 6
 non-biased, 1
Health care professionals, 1
Health examinations, periodic, 77–78
Health maintenance organizations
 (HMOs), 5
Health risks, 1
Helicobacter pylori, 51
Hematuria, 60
Hemochromatosis, 41t
Heparin, 43t
Hepatitis A
 immunization for, 76t
 prophylaxis for, 77t
Hepatitis B immunization, 76t
Herniation compressing spinal
 nerves, 72t
Heroin abuse, 19t
Herpangina, 50t
Herpes simplex virus (HSV), 56t
Herpes zoster otiticus, 48
High-risk children, 10
History of present illness (HPI), 1
Histrionic personality, 29t
HIV. See also Acquired
 immunodeficiency virus
 biology of, 57–58
Home environment, 1
Homosexuality, 33
Hospice, 6
Hospital personnel, 6–7
Hospitalization
 for anorexia and bulimia, 18
 for mania, 22
 psychiatric criteria for, 20
 for psychotic disorders, 24
Hospitals, 5
Hot & Cold theory, 4
Human bite, 46t
Human papillomavirus (HPV), 57t
Hydroxyurea, 59
Hyperactivity, 16
Hyperbaric oxygen, 42t
Hyperlipidemia, screening for, 78
Hypersomnia, 36–37
Hypertensive crisis, 22t

Hypochondriasis, 32
Hypothalamic deficiency, 66
Hypothyroidism, 40t
Hysterectomy, 66
Hysterosalpingogram, 70

I

Ideal body weight (IBW), 38
Identification, 30
Imaginary friends, 7t
Imipramine
 for depression, 22t
 for panic disorder, 26t
 for posttraumatic stress
 disorder, 27t
Immersion burns, 11
Immunization, adult, 76t
Immunologic measurements, 38
Impotence, 61–62
Impulsive-control disorders, 34
Incidence, 81t
Independent practice association
 (IPA), 5
Infectious diarrhea, 53t
Infertility, 69–70
 causes of, 66–70
Influenza immunization, 76t
Informed consent, 79
Injury, adolescence, 13
Insect bites, 45–46t
Insomnia, 36
Intellectualization, 30
Intelligence tests, 9t
Intermediate care facilities (ICF), 6
Intermediate hospital, 5
Intermittent explosive disorder, 34
Interpreter, 4–5
 in patient-doctor communications,
 85–86, 88
Interview, 1–3
Interviewing techniques, 2t
Intestinal lymphangiectasia, 54t
Intoxication, signs and symptoms of,
 19t, 85, 88
Iodine, deficiencies and excesses of, 40t
Ipecac, syrup of
 for child poisonings, 12
 for mercury poisoning, 43t
 for theophylline poisoning, 43t
Iron
 deficiencies and excesses of, 41t
 toxicology and antidotes of, 43t
Isoniazid, 43t

J

Japanese puffer fish, 45t

K

Kaposi's sarcoma, 58–59
Keshan's disease, 41t

L

Kidney stones, 41t
Kleptomania, 34
Kwashiorkor, 41t
Laboratory studies, in nutritional
    assessment, 38
Lactase deficiency, 54t
Language
    developmental milestones of, 8t
    interpreters for, 85–86, 88
Lavage, 12
Lead toxicity, 43t
Legal issues, 78–80
Leukopenia, 40t
Licensed Practical Nurse/Licensed
    Vocational Nurse (LPN/LVN), 6
Lifestyle modifications, 51
Lipid requirements, 39
Lithium
    for cluster headache, 48t
    for mania, 22
Living will, 80
Logical thoughts, 7t
Low back pain, 70–71
    red flags for, 71, 72t
LSD, 19t
Luteinizing hormone, 62

M

Magnesium, intravenous, 43t
Major depressive disorders, 21t
Mal de ojo, 4
Mal puesto, 4
Malabsorption diarrhea, 52
Maladaptive behavior, patterns
    of, 28
Malaria, prophylaxis for, 77t
Malignant otitis externa, 49
Malingering, 30
Malnutrition
    protein, 41t
    total calorie, 41t
Malpractice, 78–79
Mania, 22
Manic depression, 21t
Marasmus, 41t
Medicaid, 6
Medical interview, 1–3
Medicare, 6
Meningococcus, prophylaxis for, 77t
Menopause, 68
    premature natural, 67
Menorrhagia, 67
Menstrual cycle, 62–63
Menstruation, irregular, 67
Mercury poisoning, 43t
Metaplasia, respiratory epithelia, 41t
Methanol, 43t

Methylphenidate, 16
Methylprednisilone, 45t
Methysergide, 48t
Metronidazole
    for infectious diarrhea, 53t, 55t
    for pelvic inflammatory
        disease, 56t
    for vaginitis, 65t
Midrin, 48t
Migraine headache
    epidemiology and characteristics
        of, 47t
    treatment of, 48t
Minerals, deficiencies and excesses of,
    40–41t
Minnesota Multiphasic Personality
    Inventory (MMPI), 9t
MMR immunization, 76t
Mollusks, toxins of, 44–45t
Monoamine oxidase inhibitors, 22t
Mononucleosis, 50t
Mood disorders
    in children and adolescents, 15–16
    diagnosis of, 23t
    signs and symptoms of, 21t
    treatments of, 22
Movement disorders, antipsychotic
    associated, 25t
Multiple personality disorder, 33
Munchausen by proxy, 31
Munchausen syndrome, 31
Mycoplasma avium-intracellulare
    complex, 59
Myopathy, 41t

N

N-acetylcysteine, 42t
Narcan, 43t
Narcissistic personality, 30t
Narcolepsy, 36
Narcotics, 35t
Naturopathy, 85, 88
Negative predictive value, 81t
Neisseria gonorrhoeae pelvic
    inflammation, 56t
Neural tube defects, 40t
Neuroleptic malignant syndrome,
    antipsychotic-associated, 25t
Neuropathy, 40t
Neurotoxic shellfish, 45t
Niacin, deficiencies and excesses
    of, 40t
Nicotine replacement, 77
Night blindness, 41t
Night terror, 37
Nightmares, 37
Nimodipine, 48t
Nitrogen balance, 38

Nocturnal penile tumescence testing, 62
Non rapid eye movement (NREM) sleep, 35, 36t
Nonmalficence, 79
  definition of, 87–88
Nortriptyline, 22t
NSAIDs
  for endometriosis, 65
  for migraine, 48t
  for tension headache, 48t
  for trigeminal neuralgia, 48t
  for uterine bleeding, 68
Nucleoside analogues, 59
Nurse-maid's elbow, 74
Nurse Practitioner, 6
Nurses, 6–7
Nurses aide, 6
Nursing homes, 5
Nutrients, deficiencies and excesses of, 40–41t
Nutrition, assessment of, 37–40
Nutritional neglect, child, 10
Nutritional requirements, calculation of, 38–39
Nutritional supplements, 39–40

O

Obsessive-compulsive disorder
  characteristics of, 30t
  diagnosis, signs and symptoms, and treatment of, 26t
Odds ratio, 81t
Olanzapine, 24t
Olecranon
  bursitis, 74–75
  fracture of, 74
Oophorectomy, 66
Open ended questions, 2t
Opioids, 43t
Opportunistic infections, AIDS-related, 58–59
Oppositional defiant disorder, 16–17
Oral contraceptive pills, 63
Organophosphate, 43t
Osmotic diarrhea, 53t
Osteomalacia, 41t
Otitis externa, 48–49
Outpatient complaints
  ear, nose, and throat, 48–50
  gastrointestinal, 50–52
  gynecologic, 62–66
  headache, 46–48
  reproductive, 66–70
  urogenital, 52–62
Ovarian dysfunction, 66–67
Ovarian sex steroids, 62

P

Ovulation, 62–63
  screening test for, 69

Pancreatitis, diarrhea with, 54t
Panic disorder, 26t
Pantothenate, deficiencies and excesses of, 40t
Pap smear, 63
Paralytic shellfish, 44t
Paranoid personality, 29t
Paraphrasing, 2t
Parasomnias, 37
Parenteral feeding, 39–40
Parkinsonism, antipsychotic-associated, 25t
Paroxetine, 22t
Past medical history (PMH), 1
Past surgical history (PSH), 1
Pasteurella infection, 46t
Patient-doctor communication, interpreter in, 4–5, 85–86, 88
Patient-doctor relationship, 1
Patient history, 1
Patient interview, 1–3
Pediatric toxicology, 13t
Pellagra, 40t
Pelvic inflammatory disease, 56t
Penicillamine, 43t
Penicillin, 54t
Penile prostheses, 62
Peptic stricture, with GERD, 52
Periodic health examinations, 77–78
Pernicious anemia, 40t
Persistent vegetative state (PVS), 80
Personality disorders
  clusters of, 28
  ego defenses and, 28–30
  general characteristics of, 28
  specific types of, 29–30t
Personality tests, 9t
Pervasive developmental disorder, 14
Pharyngitis, 50
Phencyclidine abuse, 19t
Phenelzine, 22t
Phenobarbitol, 43t
Phenytoin, 48t
Physical trauma, child, 10
Physician Assistant, 7
Physostigmine, 42t
Piaget developmental theory, 7t
Pickwickian syndrome, 37
  diagnosis and treatment of, 85, 88
Pinching, 4
Pituitary dysfunction, 66
Plummer-Vinson syndrome, 41t
Pneumococcal immunization, 76t
Pneumocystis carinii pneumonia, 59

Podophyllin, 57t
Poisonings, child, 12, 13t
Positive predictive value, 81t
Posttraumatic stress disorder, 27t
Power (1-β), 81t
Power of attorney, 80
Pralidoxime, 43t
Prealbumin serum levels, 38
Preferred provider organization
  (PPO), 5
Pregnancy, 66
Prevalence, 81t, 87–88
Preventive medicine, 75–78
Primum non nocer, 79
Progesterone, 63
  serum levels of, 69
Projection, 28
Promotility agents, 51
Prospective interventional trial, 82
Prostaglandins, 62
Prostate
  cancer screening, 76t
  hyperplasia of, 60–61
Prostatitis, 61
Protamine, 43t
Protease inhibitors, 59
Protein
  deficiencies and excesses of, 41t
  requirements for, 39
Proton pump inhibitors
  for dyspepsia, 51
  for GERD, 51
Pseudomonas infection, 48
Pseudotumor cerebri, 41t
Psychiatric disorders
  prognosis of, 20t
  signs and symptoms of, 85–86, 88
Psychiatry
  child and adolescent, 14–18
  DSM-IV classifications of, 20t
  mood disorders, 21
  principles of, 20
  treatments of, 22
Psychological tests, 9t
Psychosis, 23–25
Psychosocial support, 15
Psychotherapy
  for anorexia and bulimia, 18
  for depression, 21
  for generalized anxiety
    disorder, 27t
  for hypochondriasis, 32
  for obsessive compulsive
    disorder, 26t
  for personality disorders, 28
  for posttraumatic stress
    disorder, 27t

  for psychotic disorders, 24–25
  for Tourette's disorder, 17
Psychotic disorders
  diagnosis of, 23t
  prognosis of, 25
  treatment of, 24–25
Pyelonephritis, 55
Pyridoxine
  deficiencies and excesses of, 40t
  for isoniazid poisoning, 43t
Pyromania, 34

Q
Questions, interview, 2t
Quinidine, 43t

R
Racial diversity, 1
Radiculopathy, 71
  in low back pain, 72t
Raloxifene, 68
Ramsay Hunt syndrome, 48
Rape kits, 3
Rapid eye movement (REM) sleep,
  35, 36t
Rapid transit diarrhea, 53t
Rationalization, 30
Reaction formation, 30
5-α-Reductase inhibitor, 61
Registered Nurse, 6
Regression, 30
Relative risk, 81t
Relaxation techniques
  for generalized anxiety
    disorder, 27t
  for posttraumatic stress
    disorder, 27t
Reproductive complaints, 66–70
Reproductive endocrinology, 66–70
Respiratory training, 26t
Retinol-binding protein serum
  levels, 38
Retrospective interventional trial, 82
Retrovirus, 57–58
Reverse transcriptase, HIV, 58
Riboflavin, deficiencies and excesses
  of, 40t
RICE, 75
Rickets, 41t
Risperidone, 24t
Rorschach test, 9t
Rubbing, 4

S
Safety, in patient history, 3
Salpingitis, 69
Saxitoxin, 44t
Schizoaffective disorder, 23t
Schizoid personality, 29t
Schizophrenia

diagnosis of, 23t
  prognosis for, 25
Scombroid toxin, 44t
Scombrotoxin, 44t
Scurvy, 41t
Secretory diarrhea, 53t
Sedatives, 35t
Selective serotonin reuptake
  inhibitors, 22t
Selenium, deficiencies and excesses
  of, 40t
Semen, normal, 69
Sensitivity, 82
  definition of, 81t, 87–88
Separation anxiety, 7t, 15–16
Serotonin syndrome, 22t
Sexual abuse, 11
  child, 10
Sexual activity
  in adolescents, 14
  patient history of, 3
Sexual identity disorders, 33
Sexual orientation, 33
Sexually transmitted diseases (STDs), 55
  in adolescents, 14
  characteristics and treatment of,
    56–57t
Shellfish toxins, 44–45t
Shoulder dislocation, 71–73
Sildenafil (Viagra), 62
Silence, in interview, 2t
Sinusitis, 49–50
Skilled nursing facilities, 5
Sleep
  normal, 35
  stages of, 36t
Sleep apnea, 36–37
Sleep disturbances, 16, 36–37
Sleep spindles, 36t
Sleep walking, 37
Smoking cessation, 77
Snake bite, 46t
Social developmental milestones, 8t
Social history (SH), 1
Social Security Act, Medicare/Medicaid
  authorization, 6
Social Services, Department of, 3
Sodium thiosulfate, 42t
Somatization disorder, 31–32
Somatoform disorders, 30, 31–33
Somnambulism, 37
Sorcery, 4
Specificity, 82
  definition of, 81t, 87–88
Spinal stenosis, 71
  in low back pain, 72t
Spiral fracture, 11

Splitting, 28
Sports medicine complaints, 70–75
SSRIs
  for body dysmorphic disorder, 33
  for obsessive compulsive
    disorder, 26t
  for panic disorder, 26t
Staff model HMO, 5
Statistical values, calculation of, 82–83
STD deviation, 81t
Stranger anxiety, 7t
Strep throat, Group A, 50t
Study types, 82
Subarachnoid hemorrhage
  diagnosis of, 48
  epidemiology and characteristics
    of, 47t
  treatment of, 48t
Sublimation, 30
Subluxation, shoulder, 71
Substance abuse, 13–14
Suicide
  adolescent, 13
  in patient history, 3
Sumatriptan
  for cluster headache, 48t
  for migraine, 48t
Susto, 4
Syphilis, 57t

Tanner stages, 9t
Tardive dyskinesia, antipsychotic-
  associated, 25t
Temporal arteritis
  diagnosis of, 47
  epidemiology and characteristics
    of, 47t
  treatment of, 48t
Temporal artery biopsy, 47
Tendinitis, 73–74
Tennis elbow, 73
Tension headache
  epidemiology and characteristics
    of, 47t
  treatment of, 48t
Terazosin, 61
Tertiary medical center, 5
Testosterone therapy, 62
Tetanus
  immunization for, 76t, 78
  prophylaxis for, 46t
Tetracycline
  for tropical sprue, 54t
  for Whipple's disease, 54t
Tetrodotoxin, 45t
Theophylline, 43t
Theta waves, 36t

Thiamine, deficiencies and excesses of, 40*t*
Thompson test, 75
Tort, 78
Total parenteral nutrition (TPN), 39
    discontinuing, 40
    monitoring of, 40
Tourette's disorder, 17
Toxicology, 42–46*t*
    pediatric, 13*t*
Toxins, 42–43*t*
Toxoplasma encephalitis, 59
Traction-countertraction techniques, 73
Transferrin serum levels, 38
Transurethral resection of prostate, 61
Tranylcypromine, 22*t*
Trauma, child, 10–12
Travel prophylaxis, 77*t*
Treatment plans, 1
Tremor, lithium-induced, 22
Treponema pallidum, 57*t*
Triceps skin fold, 38
Trichloracetic acid, 57*t*
Trichomonas vaginitis, 64, 65*t*
Trichotillomania, 34
Tricyclic antidepressants
    for depression, 22*t*
    for posttraumatic stress disorder, 27*t*
Tricyclics
    for panic disorder, 26*t*
    toxicology and antidotes of, 43*t*
Trigeminal neuralgia
    diagnosis of, 47–48
    epidemiology and characteristics of, 47*t*
    treatment of, 48*t*
Tropical sprue, 54*t*
Tumors, in low back pain, 71, 72*t*
Turner's syndrome, 67
Type I error, 81*t*
Type II error, 81*t*
Typhoid, prophylaxis for, 77*t*

U

Urinalysis, 60
Urinary tract infection (UTI), 54–55
Urogenital complaints, 54–62
Urogram, 60
Uterus, congenital anomaly of, 70

V

Vacuum-constriction devices, 62
Vaginitis, 64
    differential diagnosis of, 65*t*
Valacyclovir, 56*t*
Validation, interview, 2*t*
Valproate, 22
Valproic acid, 48*t*
Variance, 81*t*, 87–88
Varicella immunization, 76*t*
Vasoconstrictors, 49
Verapamil, 48*t*
Viagra, 62
Vitamin A, deficiencies and excesses of, 41*t*
Vitamin C, deficiencies and excesses of, 41*t*
Vitamin D, deficiencies and excesses of, 41*t*
Vitamin E, deficiencies and excesses of, 41*t*
Vitamin K
    deficiencies and excesses of, 41*t*
    for warfarin poisoning, 43*t*
Vitamins, deficiencies and excesses of, 40–41*t*

W

Warfarin, 43*t*
Wasp sting, 45*t*
Wechsler Adult Intelligence Scale – Revised (WAIS-R), 9*t*
Wechsler Intelligence Scale for Children–Revised (WISC-R), 9*t*
Wechsler Preschool and Primary Scale of Intelligence (WPPSI), 9*t*
Whipple's disease, 54*t*
Wide-Range Achievement Test (WRAT), 9*t*
Withdrawal headache
    epidemiology and characteristics of, 47*t*
    treatment of, 48*t*
Withdrawal symptoms, 19*t*

X

Xerophthalmia, 41*t*

Y

Yellow fever, prophylaxis for, 77*t*

Z

Zinc, deficiencies and excesses of, 41*t*